Diagnostic Immunology and Serology:
A Clinicians' Guide

Diagnostic Immunology and Serology: A Clinicians' Guide

J.D. Wilson and Sandra I. Simpson†*

*Associate Professor of Immunology
†Graduate Technologist
Department of Medicine, University of Auckland School of Medicine, Auckland, New Zealand

With 35 tables and 23 figures

MTP PRESS LIMITED *International Medical Publishers*

Diagnostic Immunology and Serology:
A Clinicians' Guide

Published in UK, Europe and Middle East
by MTP Press Limited
Falcon House
Lancaster
England

First Printing
ISBN 978-94-015-1128-5 ISBN 978-94-015-1126-1 (eBook)
DOI 10.1007/978-94-015-1126-1

MTP PRESS LIMITED International Medical Publishers

Foreword

Immunology as an independent discipline is just 100 years old. In the Pasteurian era, it was the direct handmaiden of medical microbiology, but with Landsteiner's discovery of the blood groups in 1901, immunology burst through into other fields. This spreading of immunology into many facets of biology and medicine has continued at an accelerating pace, particularly over these last 20 years. For the physician, immunology is a 'horizontal' specialty, breaking the confines of a single organ system and touching an enormous number of chronic diseases.

This spreading tendency of immunology is both a source of great fascination and great frustration. The research worker in immunology is delighted to be engaged at so many frontiers. The clinician who must use the new research knowledge to help the patient can easily be confused and overwhelmed. The fact that immunology is poorly taught in most medical courses makes things worse. These are the reasons why physicians, clinical pathologists and undergraduate and postgraudate students should hail the publication of 'Diagnostic Immunology and Serology'.

Douglas Wilson and Sandra I. Simpson have achieved a triumph in not only marrying the microbiological and general aspects of diagnostic immunology, but also in achieving an authoritative synthesis in a brief, down-to-earth, eminently readable format. Their book is not a list of recipes — it does not seek to describe the details of the various diagnostic tests used by the clinical pathologist specialising in immunology. Nor is it an erudite treatise of theoretical immunology — we have enough of those. Rather, it sets out the major immunological diagnostic techniques, describes their scientific rationale and gives the clinician a clear indication of the meaning of a positive test, all with a commendable absence of immunological jargon. The book, read cover to cover, serves as a useful guide to those aspects of modern immunology that the clinician most needs to know, and read piecemeal for specific tests, will help a physician to interpret a particular result received from the laboratory with greater perception.

As a subspecialty of clinical pathology, diagnostic immunology is relatively new. This book elegantly fills an important gap. It is a pleasure to recommend it to what I hope will be a wide readership.

G.J.V. Nossal
Director, Walter and Eliza Hall Institute, Melbourne

Preface

The rapid progress of basic immunology in recent years has been followed by a similar expansion in clinical immunology with the recognition of the immune pathogenesis of a number of diseases and the development of a wide range of laboratory assays. Commercial development of antisera, immunodiffusion plates, haemagglutination and radioimmunoassay kits has made relatively sophisticated assays available to most laboratories. While many text books on clinical immunology discuss basic immunology, immunopathogenic mechanisms and clinical features of immunologically related diseases, there is usually a lack of emphasis on the clinical immunological tests and their interpretation. This book is intended to fill that gap by providing a ready reference for the more common immunological and serological tests, with a clear guide to their interpretation. A minimum of space is given to clinical descriptions but some laboratory details of the assays are included to clarify their clinical significance. Finally, an appendix is provided as a precis of the immunological tests of relevance to the diagnosis and management of non-infectious disease.

The book was conceived by John McKay and ourselves and he has contributed much of the material for the chapters on Toxoplasmosis, Leptospirosis, Brucellosis, Hydatids, Syphilis and Acute Phase Proteins. The chapter on Neutrophil Function Tests was written by Cliff Hosking. We have taken liberties with their texts and are responsible for the final presentation, and the errors.

Our thanks are due to Mrs Norma Turner for secretarial assistance, and to Mr David Bree, Dr Ian Simpson, Mr Denis Harding, Dr Lindsay Green of Auckland, and Professor Tony Basten of Sydney for reviewing sections of the manuscript and offering valuable criticisms.

J.D. Wilson
Sandra I. Simpson
Auckland

Contributors

Wilson, J.D.
Associate Professor of Immunology, Department of Medicine, University of Auckland School of Medicine, Auckland, New Zealand.

Simpson, Sandra I.
Graduate Technologist, Department of Medicine, Section of Immunology, University of Auckland School of Medicine, Auckland, New Zealand.

McKay, E.J.
Research Fellow, Department of Clinical Chemistry, University of Lund, Malmo, Sweden.

Hosking, C.S.
Immunologist, Royal Children's Hospital, Melbourne, Australia.

Contents

Section 2: Immunological Tests

Section 3: Disease and the Immune System

Chapter I

General Principles

The assays discussed in the succeeding chapters of this book are used:

1) To evaluate the competence of the immune system itself
2) To measure a patient's immune response against foreign or self proteins (antigens)
3) To identify components of hypersensitivity reactions producing disease.

1. The Immune System

The immune system consists of specialised cells and various humoral factors such as immunoglobulins and complement. The central cells in the system are lymphocytes which either circulate between blood and lymph nodes, or are aggregated into specialised units such as the spleen, lymph nodes, tonsils and Peyers's patches. During fetal life developing lymphocytes follow one of two major pathways of differentiation, forming T and B lymphocytes. The T cells are processed in the thymus and then seed to peripheral lymphoid tissues where they serve a number of roles, from regulation of the immune response to direct cytotoxicity. B cells develop within the bone marrow before seeding to peripheral lymphoid tissue where their ultimate task is to differentiate into plasma cells and produce antibodies.

A number of other cells also participate in the immune system, either within lymph nodes or within the reticuloendothelial tissues. Neutrophils and macrophages function as phagocytic cells with the macrophages also interacting with lymphocytes in the development of immune responses. Eosinophils are involved in some antigen-antibody reactions and possibly also in phagocytosis and other scavenging operations Mast cells provide a package of inflammatory substances which, if released inappropriately, gives rise to some allergic symptoms such as urticaria or bronchospasm.

Identification and measurement of the functional integrity of most of the components of the immune system is now possible. Lymphocyte populations can be recognised and some of their *in vivo* activities can be examined *in vitro*. The competence of neutrophils is detected by various neutrophil function assays. Measurement of patients' immunoglobulins and selected complement components have now, with the development of commercially available immunodiffusion plates, become routine procedures, particularly in the consideration of various forms of immune deficiency or in measuring the aggressiveness of some antibody reactions.

2. The Immune Response

An immune response to an antigen has a number of different components and evaluation of these can provide a wide range of diagnostic information. Both T and B lymphocytes can become effector cells, the former playing a role in cell-mediated immune responses and the B cells and plasma cells secreting immunoglobulin to provide humoral immunity. Generation of an immune response following interaction with antigen is a complicated process. Interactions between various lymphocyte populations, macrophages and secreted factors produce a potent defence response which acts rapidly and selectively. A complex system of regulation limits the duration of the immune reaction and helps protect innocent bystander cells from damage. Breakdown of the regulating process can sometimes lead to host tissue damage and disease.

Under most circumstances the first component of an antibody response is IgM which rapidly declines as IgG antibody develops and this can persist for months or years. Thus demonstration that an IgM antibody against a particular organism is present in a patient's serum usually implies that contact with that organism is recent. Some, but not all, antibodies will fix complement, so analysis of complement-fixing antibodies can give precise clues to the stage of a patient's disease. The presence of antibody against an infectious organism means the patient has had contact with that organism but not necessarily that he is suffering, or has suffered, from clinical infection. The changing levels of antibody, or analysis of the different components of antibody response, are usually able to provide clear information as to present or past infection.

The cell-mediated response depends upon the production of cytotoxic T cells and various factors secreted from lymphocytes (lymphokines) which potentiate the inflammatory process. Antibody is not involved in this response. Measurement of cell-mediated responses is difficult *in vitro* except in specialised laboratories. However, delayed hypersensitivity skin tests such as the Mantoux test will demonstrate *in vivo* a patient's cell-mediated immune reactivity to injected antigens.

3. Hypersensitivity Reactions

On some occasions the immune system can actively damage its own host cells either because the immune responses are too violent, poorly regulated and disrupt surrounding tissue, or because the immune responses are misdirected against self antigens. Gell and Coombs have devised a classification for the hypersensitivity reactions damaging self tissue.

Type I: Immediate Hypersensitivity

IgE antibodies are bound to mast cell surfaces. The union of two adjacent IgE molecules with an antigen such as protein from pollen, provokes release of a number of vasoactive amines from the mast cell granules with consequent intensive local inflammation. The site of this local inflammation dictates the site of the allergic symptoms, and if this occurs in the nose it is manifest as hayfever, in the bronchi as asthma, or in the skin as urticaria.

Type II: Cytotoxic Antibody

Under some circumstances antibody is directed against self components, uniting with these with resultant tissue damage, either by lysis of host cells, by phagocytosis, or by promotion of inflammation. When the antibody is directed against red cells, autoimmune haemolytic anaemia develops, and if the antibody binds to the basement membrane of kidneys then Goodpasture's syndrome results.

Type III: Immune Complex or Arthus Reaction

When antibody is bound to antigen in some ratios it leads to the formation of immune complexes which are not readily removed by the phagocytic cells of the reticuloendothelial system, but rather tend to adhere to endothelial surfaces or basement membranes, initiating intense local inflammatory reactions. Immune complex formation provides the explanation for many pathological changes in a number of diseases including many infections, some forms of glomerulonephritis, polyarteritis, and systemic lupus erythematosus.

Type IV: Cell-Mediated Reactions

Under some circumstances a pure cell-mediated immune reaction is either misdirected against self components or is aimed at extrinsic compounds which have bound to self protein. When this occurs in the skin the phenomenon of contact dermatitis results, with a cell-mediated immune reaction directed against a combination of the sensitising agent and skin proteins.

Chapter II

Antistreptococcal Antibodies

Identification of streptococcal infections is important, largely in relation to the differential diagnosis of carditis and glomerulonephritis. Symptoms suggestive of rheumatic fever or post streptococcal glomerulonephritis require laboratory investigation to establish the patient's recent infection with streptococci. Antistreptococcal antibodies rise following infection so, when infection has terminated and bacterial cultures are negative, a diagnosis can still be made on the antibody response alone.

1. Clinical Conditions Associated with Streptococcal Infection

Antistreptococcal antibody assays should be requested wherever there is a clinical suspicion of acute glomerulonephritis or rheumatic fever.

1.1 Acute Glomerulonephritis (AGN)

Although figures vary widely from epidemic to epidemic, a small percentage of patients seem to develop acute glomerulonephritis after a β-haemolytic streptococcal infection. Acute nephritis follows a streptococcal infection within 10 days in most patients, whereas rheumatic fever has a much longer latent period — 18 days. In patients who develop high antistreptolysin-O (ASO) titres after streptococcal infections the incidence of AGN is greater than among those without high antibody titres.

The incidence of glomerulonephritis is greatest between the ages of 3 and 7 years but it can develop in children below the age of 2; in contrast, rheumatic fever rarely affects children under 2 years of age. Some adults get the disease, but the brunt of the attacks fall on school age and pre-school age children. Males are affected twice as commonly as females. 80% of the patients have a preceding upper respiratory tract infection but a few have skin infections such as impetigo. A proportion of cases occur without any apparent preceding infection and it has been suggested that in these the infection precipitating the attack of acute nephritis may be viral in origin. It is difficult to be certain about the absence of a preceding streptococcal infection unless very strict care is taken to perform all the antibody tests repeatedly, as well as taking cultures of the appropriate areas of the patient.

1.2 Rheumatic Fever

A significant proportion of patients with untreated epidemic exudative streptococcal pharyngitis develop rheumatic fever. In patient groups treated with antibiotics, rheumatic fever usually occurs only among those patients in whom the treatment fails to eradicate the streptococci. Moreover, the attack rate of rheumatic fever is decreased significantly by eradication of the streptococci as long as 9 days after the onset of symptoms, by which time maximum antibody stimulation has already occurred (Cantanzaro et al., 1954). These observations indicate that persistence of the organism in the host is critically important for the development of rheumatic fever.

The attack rate of rheumatic fever following streptococcal infections is much higher in patients who have already had rheumatic fever than in those who have not. The rate is highest in the first few months after the rheumatic attack and declines thereafter. Rheumatic fever recurrences occur only among those patients who develop a streptococcal antibody response. In those patients with antibody responses the recurrence rate per infection increases with the magnitude of the antibody rise and ranges from 15% in infections characterised by the minimum significant ASO rise to 70% in infections characterised by the maximum antibody rise observed.

Low antibody titres may be detected in patients who present with Sydenham's chorea, probably due to a longer latent period of this manifestation. Lower titres can occur in isolated cases of carditis which may have come to medical attention relatively late in their course.

Deceptively high titres may be due to non-antibody inhibitors of streptolysin-O in hepatitis, biliary obstruction and nephrotic syndrome or to monoclonal IgG in myeloma.

2. Diagnosis

Rheumatic fever and glomerulonephritis are suspected by their clinical presentation and history (table I). Establishment of recent streptococcal infection depends firstly on identification of the organism from throat or skin swabs and secondly and most commonly by serological tests.

During their growth, Group A β-haemolytic streptococci produce a number of extracellular products and enzymes which are antigenic and these promote the

Table I. Comparison between glomerulonephritis and rheumatic fever. Adapted from Youmans et al. (1973) with permission of the authors and editors

Feature	Glomerulonephritis	Rheumatic fever
Age distribution	Can affect any age	Unusual in infancy
Familial factors	Family contacts	Familial tendency
Sex distribution	Predominantly male	No difference
Incidence (following streptococcal infection)	Variable (up to 28%)	Variable (3%)
Subsequent attacks	Rare: may occur after skin infections	Relatively common
Average latent period between infection and first attack	10 days	18 days
Latent period between subsequent infection and exacerbation	Shortened compared with latent period in first attack	Same as latent period in first attack
Relation between degree of ASO increase and incidence of first attack	No relation	Incidence proportional to degree of ASO increase
Time of ASO increase in relation to onset of relapse	After	Before
Serum whole complement and C3	Decreased	Increased
M-types of initiating Group A haemolytic streptococcus	Pharyngeal: 1, 4, 12, 18 Skin: 2, 31, 49, 52-55, 57,60	Any pharyngeal type (skin strains are not rheumatogenic)

development of antibodies by the patient (fig. 1). The respective antibodies block specific enzymatic activity and thus a reduction in activity of a standard enzyme preparation can be used as an indicator for the antibody.

A battery of antistreptococcal antibody assays is necessary to confirm infection in most cases because:

a) Infecting streptococcal organisms vary
b) Different patients produce different patterns of antibody to the same organism.

A single determination of antistreptococcal antibodies is of limited value as results above the normal range may not necessarily indicate recent infection. Antibody titres are elevated for up to 4 to 6 weeks after infection, so serial tests are necessary to detect this rise. Titres will decline very slowly over 6 months. When titres do not fall, the possibility of recurrent infection must be considered.

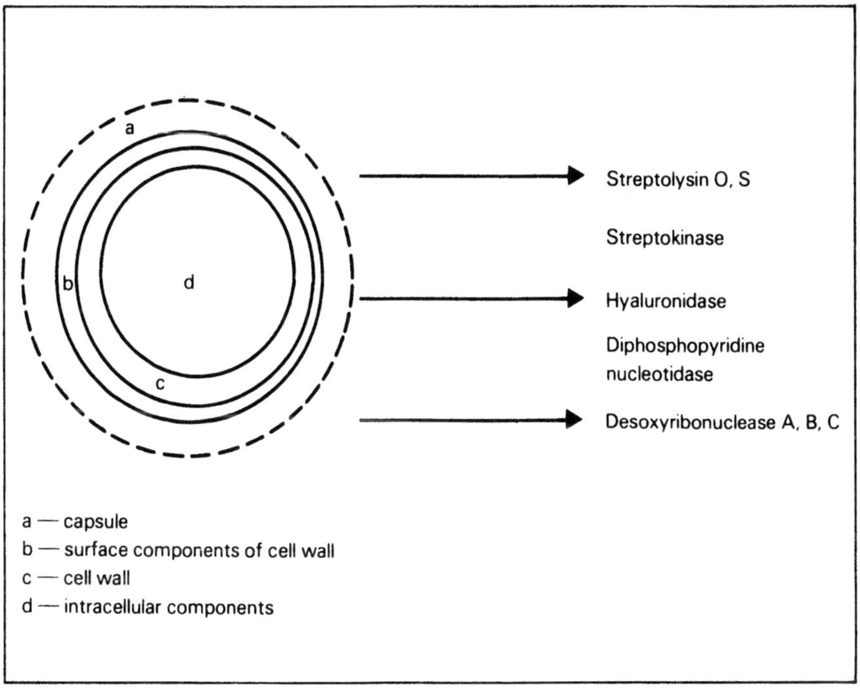

Fig. 1. Diagrammatic representation of the cellular structure and some of the antigenic extracellular products of group A streptococci (adapted with permission of the authors from Wannamaker and Ayoub, 1960).

A single assay, even if used serially, will not detect all patients reacting to streptococcal infection but with multiple tests most patients will be diagnosed. 60 to 80% of Group A streptococcal infections are detected by antistreptolysin O (ASO) alone, about 80 to 90% when both ASO and antihyaluronidase (AHT) are used, and 95% when antistreptokinase (ASK) is estimated in addition.

3. Individual Antibody Assays

3.1 Antistreptolysin-O Test (ASO)

Group A streptococci produce a haemolytic factor, streptolysin-O, which is capable of haemolysing red blood cells. The release of streptolysin-O during an infection stimulates the development of specific antistreptolysin-O antibodies. When a patient's serum containing this antibody is added to streptolysin *in vitro* an antigen-antibody reaction will occur, antistreptolysin neutralising the streptolysin, in part or completely, depending on the concentration of antibody. This reaction is visualised and measured by addition of red cells to various titres of serum.

Evaluation of the ASO Titre [Normal level less than 300 international units (iu)/ml]

Group A streptococcal infections are common, especially in school-aged children, and significant levels of antistreptococcal antibodies are found in healthy individuals. The new born child has titres similar to the mother but they fall significantly by 6 months of age. Streptococcal infections are uncommon under 2 years of age and children in this age group usually have ASO titres less than 50 iu/ml. School-aged children, particularly in the 5 to 12 year age group, are repeatedly exposed to streptococci and often have ASO titres of up to 300iu/ml in the absence of recent infection. In adults the upper limit of normal is slightly lower, about 125iu/ml. This same pattern is seen with all the antistreptococcal antibodies.

In adults the accepted upper limit of normal for the ASO test is considered to be 200iu/ml. Titres of 300iu/ml or more, rising over 2 to 4 weeks, indicate infection. It must be remembered that rising titres indicate β-haemolytic streptococcal infection and not necessarily rheumatic fever or acute glomerulonephritis.

Deceptively high titres may be due to non-antibody inhibitors of streptolysin-O as in hepatitis, biliary obstruction and conditions with high cholesterol levels or with myeloma protein. Low ASO titres may be found in patients with immunoglobulin deficiencies. Patients with non-suppurative complications of streptococcal infections (e.g. acute rheumatic fever and acute glomerulonephritis) have a higher incidence of elevated ASO titres (80 *vs* 60%) and higher numerical titres, than patients with uncomplicated streptococcal disease (Glynn, 1975). An important exception to this is in streptococcal pyoderma in which few individuals (25%) demonstrate an elevated ASO titre even if acute glomerulonephritis occurs.

3.2 Antihyaluronidase Test (AHT)

This test is based on the inhibition of streptococcal hyaluronidase by antihyaluronidase in the patient's serum. Excess hyaluronidase is measured by its ability to hydrolyse potassium hyaluronate. The antihyaluronidase titre is the reciprocal of the highest serum dilution showing a clot *in vitro*. The antibody titre of hyaluronidase rises in the second week after infection and falls in 3 to 5 weeks.

Evaluation of the AHT (Normal levels less than 1 : 500)

AHT shows elevated titres in approximately 60% of streptococcal respiratory tract infections.

By itself the AHT is less helpful than the ASO titre but when they are used in association, 80 to 90% of persons with an antecedent streptococcal respiratory infection will show an elevated titre to at least one of the antigens. Healthy people may exhibit titres of up to 1 : 500 and following infection titres of greater than 1 : 1000 are frequently seen.

3.3 Antistreptokinase Test (ASK)

This test is prepared by using a mixture of streptokinase and streptodornase which has been absorbed onto previously fixed sheep red cells. Addition of serum containing antistreptokinase antibody produces agglutination of the red cells. The antibody level can then be titred.

Evaluation of the ASK Titre (Normal levels are 1 : 640 or below)

The rise in antistreptokinase titre following a streptococcal infection, with or without complications, follows the same general pattern as the ASO titre although studies show that antibody responses occur less frequently to streptokinase. Titres of 1 : 1000 or more are common after infection. ASK values are not affected by hypercholesterolaemia.

3.4 Deoxyribonuclease Test (Anti-DNAse-B)

To determine anti-DNAse-B titres, the patient's serum is inactivated to remove its own DNAse and then diluted and added to standard amounts of antigen. After incubation a DNA substrate is added to each tube and a dye is used as an indicator of remaining intact DNA.

Highly polymerised DNA forms a mucin-like clot and the presence of a clot indicates inhibition of the enzyme DNAse-B (i.e. presence of antibody). Results are read as a colour change in the dye and are expressed as a titre.

Evaluation of the Anti-DNAse B Test (Titres of up to 250 units are found in normal subjects)

In patients with rheumatic fever about 80 % of cases show raised anti-DNAse-B titres and some workers find this figure corresponds to results obtained using the ASO test.

In glomerulonephritis following streptococcal pyoderma 60 % of patients have a positive anti-DNAse test but only about 25 % have elevated ASO titres (Bisno and Ofek, 1974). Some workers have found AHT and ASK are raised more frequently than ASO in patients with pyoderma. As yet no comparison between anti-DNAse-B and ASK or AHT in pyoderma is available. In contrast, when glomerulonephritis follows streptococcal pharyngitis, about 75 % of patients show elevated anti-DNAse-B. If this test is performed in conjunction with other antistreptococcal antibody assays, evidence of glomerulonephritis following streptococcal pyoderma is more frequently obtained.

3.5 Streptozyme Test

This test utilises a standardised suspension of aldehyde-fixed sheep cells sensitised with streptococcal exoenzymes: streptolysin, streptokinase, deoxyribonuclease-B (or streptodornase) and nicotinamide adenine dinucleotidase. The test is performed by mixing a dilution of the serum to be examined with a drop of the streptozyme. Agglutination is an indication of a positive result.

Evaluation of the Streptozyme Test

This test can be considered to be a rapid combination test in that a number of antibodies are tested for simultaneously. Approximately 80% of the sera positive by the streptozyme test have an ASO titre of 160 or over, while an additional 10% show an ASK and/or AHT titre also above 160. Positive agglutination in the case of the other 10% is considered to be due to the presence of antibodies to other streptococcal enzymes or to the combined effect of several antibodies which individually would fall below the 160 titre.Practically no sera with an elevated ASO titre can be missed by the streptozyme slide test. Cholesterol and β-lipoproteins which may cause positive titres with the classical ASO test do not interfere with the streptozyme test. A full careful evaluation of this assay is still awaited.

4. Further Diagnostic Features of Rheumatic Fever

1) The ESR is elevated and the C-reactive protein (CRP) test is positive in virtually all patients with recent untreated rheumatic fever with the exception of those presenting with chorea only.

The CRP test reverts to normal before the ESR. In some patients the ESR remains elevated for a very long time in the absence of other evidence of disease. The elevated ESR of rheumatic fever is traditionally considered to be decreased by congestive heart failure but it is usually not decreased to normal levels since in a series of patients with episodes of congestive heart failure closely associated with other clinical manifestations of rheumatic fever, the ESR was consistently high.

2) The serum concentrations of gammaglobulins, alpha-2 globulins (haptoglobulins and alpha-2 macroglobulins) mucoproteins and polysaccharides are increased while albumin concentration is decreased.

3) Plasma volume appears to be increased which may account, at least in part, for the apparent mild or moderate anaemia found in this disease.

4) Patients with rheumatic fever may also have anti-heart antibodies.

5. Further Diagnostic Features of Acute Glomerulonephritis

1) Antistreptococcal antibody titres are usually, but not invariably, elevated and as the elevation may be transient, and is sometimes delayed for some weeks, tests should be repeated several times in suspicious cases if negative results are obtained. The use of antibiotics may suppress the antibody response so the absence of a positive titre does not exclude a streptococcal infection in patients receiving antibiotics.

2) The haemoglobin level is depressed in about half the patients because of the increased plasma volume, but many patients have no anaemia at all.

3) The leukocyte count is normal unless the patient is still suffering from the precipitating infection.

4) The ESR is usually elevated unless congestive heart failure is present.

5) Complement fraction C3 falls to a very low level in most patients. Serum anticomplementary activity is frequently present. Rising complement levels herald recovery.

References

Bisno, A.L. and Ofek, I.: Serologic diagnosis of streptococcal infection. American Journal of Diseases of Children 127: 676-681 (1974).

Cantanzaro, F.J.; Stetson, C.A.; Morris, A.J.; Chamowitz, R.; Rammelkamp, C.H.; Stolzer, B.L. and Perry, W.D.: The role of the streptococcus in the pathogenesis of rheumatic fever. American Journal of Medicine 17: 749-756 (1954).

Glynn, L.E.: Rheumatic fever; in Gell, Coombs and Lachmann (Eds) Clinical Aspects of Immunology. 3rd Edition p.1079-1098 (Blackwell, Oxford 1975).

Wannamaker, L.W. and Ayoub, E.M.: Antibody titres in acute rheumatic fever. Circulation 21: 598-614 (1960).

Youmans, G.P.; Paterson, P.Y. and Sommers, H.M.: The Biologic and Clinical Basis of Infectious Diseases, p.212-232 (Saunders, Philadelphia, 1973).

Further Reading

Dillon, H.C. Jr. and Reeves, M.S.A.: Streptococcal immune response in neprhitis after skin infection. American Journal of Medicine 56: 333-346 (1974).

Gaedvalk -de Grost, L.E.; Michel-Bensink, N.; von Es-Boon, M.M.; von Vonno, A.H. and Michel, M.F.: Comparison of the titres of ASO, anti DNAse B and antibodies against the group polysaccharide of group A streptococci in children with streptococcal infection. Journal of Clinical Pathology 27: 801-896 (1974).

Gell, Coombs and Lachman (Eds): Clinical Aspects of Immunology, 3rd Edition (Blackwell, Oxford 1975).

Silverman, B.K.; Bierman, R.H.; Atkin, D.; Katz, N.S.; Janeff, J.D. and Janeff, D.G.: Comparative serological changes following treated group A streptococcal pharyngitis. American Journal of Diseases of Children 127: 498-501 (1974).

Chapter III

Brucellosis

Human brucellosis is not a common disease. It is transmitted to man from animals such as cattle, pigs and goats. Man contracts the disease directly from infected animals, contaminated secretions or excretions and products of conception, the latter being particularly hazardous. Organisms invade through small abrasions of the skin or by the ingestion of raw milk by the host. Because of the danger to public health, the general population nowadays is protected by compulsory pasteurisation of milk destined for human consumption, with the result that human brucellosis is now primarily an occupational disease.

Brucella abortus is the prime infecting organism and usually produces a milder disease than *Br. suis* or *Br. melitensis.* Direct contact with infected cattle is the likeliest cause of infection; therefore farmers, slaughterhouse workers, butchers and especially veterinarians are at risk. Agricultural engineers, meat processing maintenance workers and families of dairy farmers are also potentially at risk as infection can occur from contaminated implements. Brucellosis in children does occur but is much less frequent than in adults.

1. Clinical Features

Human brucellosis is a debilitating disease and presents in three forms:

1) Acute brucellosis
2) Chronic brucellosis following an acute attack
3) Chronic brucellosis of insidious onset.

The incubation period in acute brucellosis is usually short (5-21 days) but may occasionally be as long as 6 to 9 months. Often the disease may have an abrupt onset, presenting with fatigue, severe headaches, fluctuating temperatures with drenching sweats and general malaise. These symptoms make it difficult to distinguish brucellosis from other febrile conditions, particularly leptospirosis and toxoplasmosis.

Table I. Examples of typical antibody levels in brucellosis

Type of infection	Test[1]		
	SAT	AG	CFT
Acute brucellosis	320	640	256
	80	320	16
	1280	10240	1024
Chronic brucellosis	40	160	16
	20	160	2
	40	320	16
Treated brucellosis	40	80	Nil
	40	160	2

1 SAT: slide agglutination test. AG: antiglobulin test. CFT: complement fixation test.

The onset of chronic brucellosis may be insidious or may present as an acute relapse long after an assumed cure. There is commonly a history of recurring 'flu'-like symptoms.

2. Diagnosis

A history of possible exposure to the disease coupled with symptoms consistent with brucellosis should lead the physician to make a presumptive diagnosis which should be followed by relevant laboratory tests.

The diagnosis of brucellosis can only be made absolute when the infecting organism is isolated from blood culture or tissue. The rate of isolation of brucellosis in humans is very low; therefore laboratory diagnosis rests heavily on serological findings.

3. Laboratory Tests

The serological results depend on the clinical form and stage of the disease. Clinical details are frequently not given, making laboratory diagnosis more difficult. Simple agglutination tests alone are no longer sufficient and detection of all types of antibodies involved is often necessary. In the acute stage of the disease there is the initial production of IgM antibodies followed closely by IgG. Chronic brucellosis shows a predominance of IgG and IgA antibodies with little or no IgM present.

The serological tests available are:

1) Rapid slide agglutination screen
2) Standard agglutination test
3) The antiglobulin or Coombs' test
4) The complement fixation test
5) The indirect fluorescent test.

3.1 The Rapid Slide Screen

A concentrate of whole brucella organisms is added to undiluted fresh serum, mixed for 4 minutes, macroscopic clumping being observed in positive cases. Any positive screen test should be tested further by other methods. This test will adequately detect acute brucellosis cases but may be negative with chronic brucellosis.

3.2 Standard Agglutination Test

A standard *Br. abortus* suspension is added to serial dilutions of the test serum. Dilutions ranging from 1 : 20 through to 1 : 1200 are well mixed with antigen and incubated for 18 to 24 hours at 37°C. The amount of macroscopic clumping is compared with a known standard serum. The antibody level is recorded as the highest dilution of serum in which agglutination takes place. Caution must be taken to avoid prozone phenomena caused by excessive antibody which may lead to false negative results in low titre. Primarily this test detects IgM antibodies.

3.3 Antiglobulin Test (Coombs' Test)

This test is capable of detecting the three major classes of antibody observed in brucellosis. Once the standard agglutination test is read, the same tubes are used for the antiglobulin reaction. The suspension in the test series is washed three times in isotonic saline. Suitably diluted anti-human globulin is added to each tube. Tubes are then mixed vigorously, left standing for 5 minutes and centrifuged at high speed (3400 RPM) for 60 seconds. Presence of macroscopic agglutination denotes a positive result.

3.4 Complement Fixation Test

This is one of the most important single tests available. To serial dilutions of test serum is added a known concentration of *Br. abortus* antigen, followed by a standard amount of guinea pig complement. The mixtures are incubated for 60 minutes at 37°C. Sheep red cells sensitised with rabbit haemolytic antibody are added to each test dilution, mixed and incubated for a further 30 minutes at 37°C. The antibody level is expressed as the reciprocal of the highest dilution of serum that produces 50% lysis of the sheep red cells.

3.5 Indirect Fluorescent Test

A standard concentrate of *Br. abortus* is spotted onto a microscope slide and allowed to air dry. Dilutions of test serum are applied to individual antigen areas and these are incubated at 37°C for 30 minutes in a moist chamber, then washed three times for a period of 10 minutes. The slides are then flooded with fluorescein-conjugated anti-human serum, incubated for a further 30 minutes, washed, dried and mounted in buffered glycerol. A positive result is denoted by the presence of brightly fluorescing organisms.

4. Evaluation of Tests

Acute brucellosis presents little problem as in most cases agglutination and complement fixation tests show high antibody levels, reaching a peak and gradually declining over a period of 12 months. Agglutination titres of 1 : 160 or more, antiglobulin levels 1 : 320 or more and complement fixation levels of at least 1 : 16 are generally seen.

If there has been inadequate treatment and infection does not resolve spontaneously, a state of chronic brucellosis may occur with localising of phagocytosed brucellae in various parts of the body. Liberation of organisms after breakdown of phagocytes will cause a recurrence of symptoms with an antibody pattern similar to the later stages of acute infection.

Chronic brucellosis usually presents with a negative agglutination screen and an absent or low agglutination titre. Antiglobulin and complement fixation tests however are usually strongly positive (1 : 160 and 1 : 16 respectively). Symptoms may persist long after serological evidence has disappeared.

Table I illustrates typical antibody levels found in cases of brucellosis.

5. False Positive and Negative Results

Progress in response to treatment can not always be judged from serial antibody levels as these may remain positive long after an effective cure and high levels of circulating IgG antibodies may be found without any active disease (e.g. symptomless veterinarians often have very high antibody levels). Conversely negative serology can be seen in subjects with active symptomatic disease. Fortunately this is rare for most tests will become clearly positive in 2 to 3 weeks.

Further Reading

Buchanan T.M.; Sulzer, C.R.; Frix, M.K. and Feldman, R.A.: Brucellosis in the United States, 1960-1972. An abattoir associated disease Part II. Diagnostic aspects. Medicine 53: 415-425 (1974).

Henderson, R.J.; Hill, D.M.; Vickers, A.F.; Edwards, J.M.B. and Tiller, H.E.: Brucellosis and veterinary surgeons. British Medical Journal 2: 656-659 (1975).

Chapter IV

Leptospirosis

Leptospirosis is a disease caused by the spiral bacterium *Leptospira*. It is principally a septicaemic infection with clinical symptoms that vary widely. The severity of the disease is due partly to the infecting strain and partly to the physical condition of the host. The diagnosis of leptospirosis on clinical grounds alone is unreliable and it is necessary to have laboratory confirmation, either by isolating the pathogen, or more commonly, from specific serological evidence.

Human infections usually occur sporadically, with climatic and environmental factors playing a vital role in survival of these pathogenic organisms. Moisture, warmth and a neutral pH of soil and water most favour the survival of pathogenic leptospires, spring and summer months having the highest incidence.

Leptospira is transmitted from reservoir host to man by either direct or indirect contact. Direct contact usually involves handling of reservoir hosts or their carcasses; indirect contact is by infected blood, tissues, organs or urine.

The site of entry for the organisms is via the skin, nose or muzzle (especially of grazing animals), mouth or conjunctiva. The principle reservoir hosts are cattle, rats, mice, birds and hedgehogs. Many pathogenic serotypes have been isolated — e.g. *L. icerohaemorraghiae*, *L. hebdomadis*, *L. ballum*, *L. pomona* and *L. tarassovi*.

1. Clinical Features

Infection presents as an acute pyrexial illness lasting 7 to 13 days. The major clinical features are headache, conjunctivitis, anorexia and abdominal pain. Jaundice appears in many patients, the incidence varying with the infecting serotype. Haemorrhagic complications such as haemarthrosis and haemoptysis appear in very ill patients who may also develop renal failure.

Leptospiral organisms rapidly penetrate surface epithelium and reach the bloodstream without definite lesions at the site of entry or obvious regional lymphadenitis. The incubation period is about 2 to 20 days followed by fever. As leptospires are blood borne, any organ or tissue may be affected and the ultimate distribution and concentration of micro-organisms probably accounts for the many combinations of symptoms and clinical signs observed during the course of the disease.

Organisms are present in blood during the first 2 weeks of the illness and in urine from the second to the third or fourth weeks.

2. Diagnosis

A history of acute pyrexial illness with aseptic meningitis in a patient living on a farm, or associated with potentially infected animals, strongly suggests the diagnosis of leptospirosis.

The organism can be isolated from blood or urine and identified by culture. The commonest diagnostic aids are the serological assays. These include:

1) Leptospiral slide agglutination test
2) Complement fixation test
3) Microscopic agglutination test
4) Sensitised erythrocyte lysis test
5) Indirect immunofluorescence test.

Leptospira has a complex antigenic system which has not been fully elucidated. However, antigen/antibody reactions are used successfully to identify specific leptospiral strains, to diagnose current infections and follow the epidemiology of leptospirosis in man and in domestic and wild animals.

2.1 Slide Agglutination Test

This procedure uses a formalised suspension of leptospira which gives rise to macroscopic clumping when added to serum antibody.

A range of known serotypes are pooled and one drop of this suspension is mixed with one drop of undiluted test serum on a microscope slide and rotated for 4 minutes. Macroscopic agglutination is observed by indirect light over a dark background.

When correctly performed this test is a good screen for detecting current infections. Positive results can be titred using these suspensions — however microscopic agglutination titres with individual live organisms are preferable.

2.2 Complement Fixation Test

This is a standard complement fixation test with leptospira as antigen. Fixation of complement is detected using sensitised sheep red blood cells as the indicator.

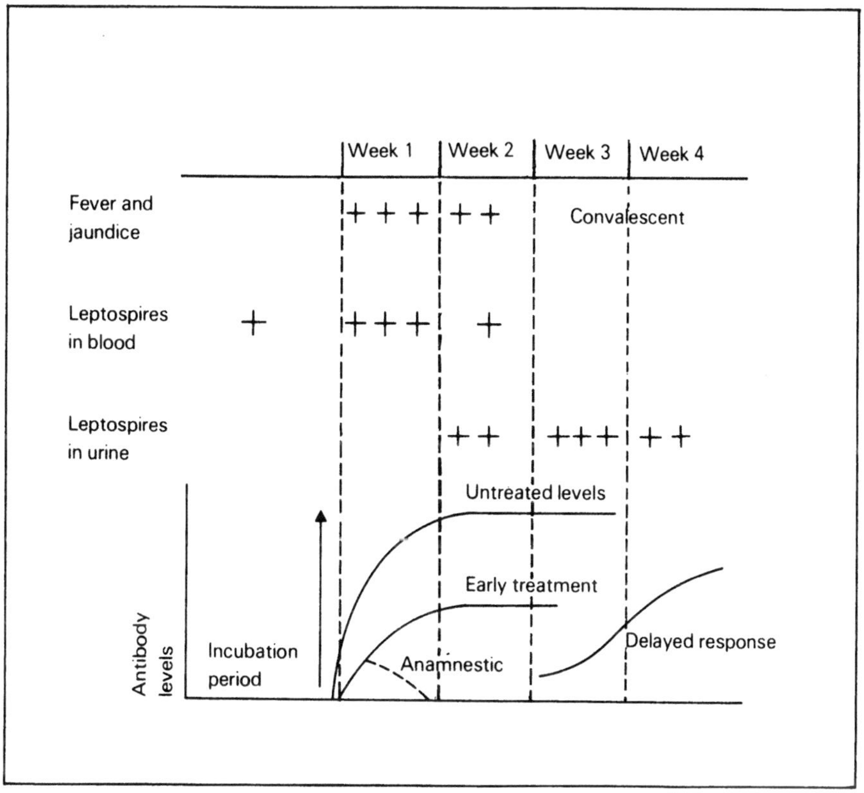

Fig. 1. Clinical and immunological signs and symptoms of leptospirosis.

This test is very useful for determining current and recently acquired infections and it shows excellent agreement with the more time-consuming microscopic agglutination test. Its disadvantage is that it is genus specific, not type specific. A pool of differing pathogenic leptospires can be used, or a single saprophytic biflexa strain (PATOC 1) is an adequate substitute.

The advantage of the complement fixation test is that it reverts to negative more quickly than other serological tests; it thus becomes possible to distinguish past from current infection and the need to maintain a constant battery of live micro-organisms is eliminated.

2.3 Microscopic Agglutination Test

Suspensions of formalised killed, or living, cultures are used in this test. To serial dilutions of test serum are added equal volumes of leptospiral suspension which agglutinate in the presence of antibody and are visualised by dark ground microscopy at 120 to 150 times magnification. The accepted end point of such an agglutination reaction is the final dilution of test serum where there are 50% of leptospires agglutinated.

To ensure adequate detection, strains known to be infecting the locality should be used, as this test is type rather than genus specific.

Formalised suspensions are less sensitive than live cultures and tend to crossreact much more, thus making serological identification of the infecting leptospiral strain more difficult.

2.4 Sensitised Lysis Test

Leptospiral antigenic material is adsorbed onto red blood cells. When these sensitised blood cells are mixed with test sera containing homologous antibody, agglutination of the red cells occurs. If complement is present lysis rather than agglutination occurs. This test appears less sensitive than the microscopic agglutination but has been used to diagnose human leptospirosis.

2.5 Indirect Immunofluorescence

In this test leptospiral organisms are spotted onto glass slides. Test serum and dilutions are added to each antigen area and incubated for 30 minutes. Washing of non-antibody protein from these slides is followed by the addition of fluorescein-labelled antiglobulin reagent. If test sera contain specific homologous antibody then leptospiral organisms will fluoresce brightly under ultraviolet light. Although little research using this test procedure has been done it appears to have a similar sensitivity to the microscopic agglutination test (McKay, personal communication).

3. Evaluation of Serological Findings

The significance of the titre/antibody level must be considered in the light of the onset of the illness. There is a rapid rise in antibody level, with a plateau of sustained high levels, followed by a slow falling of the antibody level (fig. 1). Genus specific tests, such as the complement fixation test, become positive earlier than the microscopic agglutination test and also revert to negative earlier.

Although the tests vary in sensitivity, and the height of the curve will be affected, a fourfold rise in antibody level with paired sera taken 2 to 3 weeks apart is considered almost diagnostic of current or very recent leptospirosis. The first blood sample should be taken as soon as possible after the onset of symptoms and before treatment has commenced. The later the first specimen is obtained the less likely it is that there will be a significant increase in antibody level.

A single specimen with microscopic agglutination levels of 1 : 200 or more, and complement fixation levels of 1 : 64 or more is considered fairly good evidence of recent infection.

Further Reading

Feigin, R.D. and Anderson, D.C.: Human leptospirosis. Critical Reviews in Clinical Laboratory Sciences 5: 413-467 (1975).

Chapter V

Infectious Mononucleosis

Infectious mononucleosis is normally a benign, viral disease which occurs most commonly in teenagers and young adults. It is invariably associated with the Epstein-Barr virus which is considered to be a member of the herpes virus group.

1. Clinical Features

The symptoms of the disease are usually acute and typically include headache, malaise, sore throat and fever. Exudative tonsillitis, pharyngitis and localised lymphadenopathy are very indicative of the illness. The frequency with which various signs and symptoms appear in infectious mononucleosis and their onset and duration are given in table I and figure 1.

The principal target for the virus is the lymphoid system. The Epstein-Barr virus enters B lymphocytes where it replicates, stimulating a marked and prolonged T cell response. The peripheral lymph tissue is involved, especially the tonsils, lymph nodes, spleen and liver. Lymph nodes enlarge, with great expansion of the paracortical region. Atypical lymphocytes (largely T cells) appear in the peripheral blood and it has been shown that the absolute numbers of both T and B cells can increase 5 to 10 times. Occasionally large reticulum cells with the same appearance as those found in Hodgkin's disease appear.

Other changes to be noted with the illness are reduced platelet counts, hepatomegaly and abnormal liver function tests.

Clinically the differential diagnosis includes viral or bacterial throat infections, rubella, influenza, and toxoplasmosis.

Complications can include secondary bacterial pharyngitis, neurological and haematological complications and rupture of the spleen. Fever usually subsides in the first week or two and lymphadenopathy and splenomegaly usually disappear over a

Table I. Approximate frequency of various signs and symptoms of infectious mononucleosis in young adults. From Finch (1969) with permission of the author

Symptom or sign	Percentage incidence	Symptom or sign	Percentage incidence
Adenopathy	100	Myalgia	12-30
Malaise and fatigue	90-100	Hepatomegaly	15-25
Fever	80-90	Rhinitis	10-25
Sweats	80-95	Ocular muscle pain	10-20
Sore throats, dysphagia	80-85	Chest pain	5-20
Pharyngitis	65-85	Jaundice	5-10
Anorexia	50-80	Arthralgia	5-10
Nausea	50-70	Diarrhoea or soft stools	5-10
Splenomegaly	50-60	Photophobia	5-10
Headache	40-70	Skin rash[1]	3-6
Chills	40-60	Conjunctivitis	< 5
Bradycardia	35-50	Abdominal pain	< 5
Cough	30-50	Gingivitis	< 3
Periorbital oedema	25-40	Pneumonitis	< 3
Palatal enanthem	25-35	Epistaxis	< 3
Liver or splenic tenderness	15-30		

1 Incidence of skin rash much higher when ampicillin is prescribed for treatment of this disease.

period of about 4 weeks, although lethargy and malaise may continue for a longer period. It is rare for a patient to have a recurrence of infectious mononucleosis.

2. Diagnosis

The diagnosis of infectious mononucleosis cannot be made on clinical grounds alone. When the disease is suspected tests should include a full blood count (including blood film) and a Paul-Bunnell-Davidsohn test. A throat swab is necessary to exclude bacterial infections. Assays for toxoplasmosis and rubella may be necessary.

2.1 The Paul-Bunnell-Davidsohn Test

During the course of infectious mononucleosis heterophile antibodies of the IgM class are produced. A heterophile antibody can be defined as one which reacts not only with the antigen which stimulates its production but also with biologically unrelated antigens. The classical Paul-Bunnell test has been modified because it has

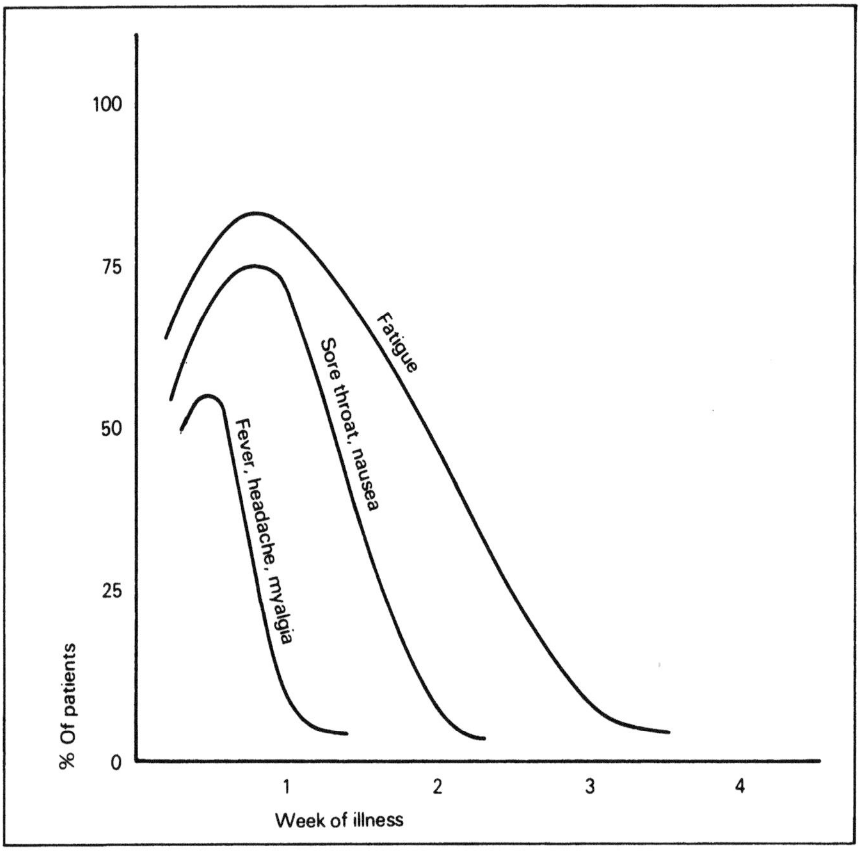

Fig. 1. Onset and duration of major symptoms of infectious mononucleosis (from Finch, 1969 [p.20] with permission of the author).

been found to fail to differentiate between the heterophile antibody of infectious mononucleosis and other heterophile antibodies such as those of the commonly occurring Forssman type and those which may occur in other illnesses such as serum sickness. The modified version of the test is called the Paul-Bunnell-Davidsohn test and is dependent on the fact that the Forssman type of agglutinins are absorbed by a suspension of guinea pig (or horse) kidney cells but not by ox cells (Davidsohn and Nelson, 1974). The reverse is true of the heterophile agglutinins of infectious mononucleosis. In brief the test depends upon the fact that the IgM antibody of infectious mononucleosis will agglutinate sheep red cells after being absorbed by preincubation with pig red blood cells. An antibody titre of over 1 : 80 is taken as positive and in infectious mononucleosis the titre usually rises after the third day of illness, reaches a maximum in about 14 days and then remains high for about 6 weeks.

Table II. Other laboratory detected abnormalities associated with infectious mononucleosis. From Finch (1969) with permission of the author and editors

Laboratory finding	Percentage incidence
Lymphocytosis, relative and absolute	100
Atypical lymphocytosis, definite[1]	100
Epstein-Barr virus (EBV) antibody in serum	100[2]
Heterophile antibody	80-100
Liver enzyme abnormalities	80-100
Leucocytosis	60-80
Neutropenia	60-80
Hyperbilirubinaemia	30-50
Bone marrow granulomata	50
Slight thrombocytopenia	25-50
Increased cell agglutinins	10-50[2]
Occult haemolysis	20-40[2]
Hyperuricaemia	15-20[2]
Leucopenia	10-20

1 20% or more of white blood cells in peripheral blood.
2 Tentative values based on scanty information.

It is considered that 90% of all patients with infectious mononucleosis show a positive Paul-Bunnell-Davidsohn test at some time (Davidsohn and Nelson, 1974). It is important that an initial negative test should be followed by a second test if symptoms are still present.

False positives can reflect an anamnestic response to a previous infection but may occur in some other diseases. Thse include aplastic anaemia, polycythaemia, agranulocytosis, splenic thrombocytopenia, thyrotoxicosis, chronic nephritis, Hodgkin's disease, myelogenous leukaemia, staphylococcal infections, sarcoma, infectious hepatitis, tuberculosis. Very high titres have been reported in acute leukaemia and serum sickness.

The diagnosis cannot therefore be solely based on a positive test and results must be considered along with other clinical and serological indications.

2.2 Monospot Test

This is a rapid slide test based on the Paul-Bunnell-Davidsohn method. It is most useful for screening purposes but can produce false positive results. A full Paul-Bunnell-Davidsohn test should always be used to confirm positive results obtained by the Monospot test.

2.3 Epstein-Barr Virus Antibody Test

A number of more complicated serological tests for Epstein-Barr virus antibodies have been used to a limited extent. Some Epstein-Barr virus specific antibodies are only transient and at present the heterophile agglutinin test remains the most useful one for diagnosis of the acute illness.

3. Additional Laboratory Diagnostic Features

Further abnormalities associated with infectious mononucleosis which can be detected by the appropriate laboratory test are listed in table II.

References

Davidsohn, I. and Nelson D.A.: The blood; in Davidsohn and Henry (Eds) Clinical Diagnosis by Laboratory Methods, p.262-264 (Saunders, Philadelphia 1974).

Finch, S.C.: Clinical symptoms and signs of infectious mononucleosis; in Carter and Penman (Eds) Infectious Mononucleosis p.19-46 (Blackwell, Oxford 1969).

Finch, S.C.: Laboratory findings in infectious mononucleosis; in Carter and Penman (Eds) Infectious Mononucleosis p.47-62 (Blackwell, Oxford 1969).

Further Reading

Ginsburg, C.M.; Henle, W.; Henle, G. and Horwitz, C.A.: Infectious mononucleosis in children. Evaluation of Epstein-Barr virus-specific serological data. The Journal of the American Medical Association 237: 781-785 (1977).

Nye, F.J.: Problems in the diagnosis and treatment of infectious mononucleosis. The Practitioner 218: 367-370 (1977).

Chapter VI

Viral Hepatitis

Three types of virus produce acute hepatitis in man. Hepatitis A has initially been identified as the agent most commonly producing infectious hepatitis, hepatitis B as the type causing most cases of serum hepatitis, and a non-A non-B virus has very recently been implicated in both forms of hepatitis (Alter et al., 1978). Hepatitis A and B viruses have been identified morphologically by electron microscopy and by various serological tests.

A number of tests are now widely available for the identification of hepatitis B and some have been developed for hepatitis A, but their use is still restricted to research institutions. No serological tests have yet been developed for the non-A non-B hepatitis virus.

1. Clinical Features of Hepatitis A and B

Some clinical difference is seen between the two types of hepatitis. Hepatitis A is frequently heralded by nonspecific symptoms such as fever, chill, headache, fatigue, generalised weakness and aches and pains. A few days later anorexia, nausea, vomiting and right upper quadrant pain develop followed by the passage of dark urine, light stools and the development of jaundice.

The prodromal symptoms of hepatitis B are often prolonged and more insidious, with low-grade fever, arthralgias and skin rashes, usually urticarial.

The well known clinical features of the established hepatitis are similar for both type A and type B viruses. The mortality is similar for the two diseases except for hepatitis B following blood transfusions, or hepatitis A during pregnancy, when the mortality is substantially higher.

Hepatitis caused by the non-A non B-virus is not readily distinguishable from hepatitis B on clinical grounds.

2. Nomenclature

An agreed nomenclature has been published by the World Health Organisation (WHO Bulletin, 1977).

2.1 Hepatitis A Virus

Hepatitis A virus is usually termed HAV. It is a small virus with a diameter of 25 to 28nm. The antibody to HAV is termed anti-HAV.

2.2 Hepatitis B Virus

This is referred to as HBV. It is larger than HAV (about 42nm) and its original name was the Dane particle.

The surface antigen on HBV is referred to as HBsAg. This is found both on the surface of the virus and in other forms in serum or on infected cells. There is an antigen found in the core of the virus and this is referred to as HBcAg. A third antigen (HBeAg) is also closely associated with hepatitis B infection.

The antibodies to the various HBV antigens are termed anti-HBs, anti-HBc and anti-HBe.

A third type of hepatitis which has been clinically recognised does not seem to be antigenically related to HBV or HAV.

3. Diagnosis

The diagnosis of acute hepatitis is made on clinical grounds and by selected liver function assays. The serological tests are used to establish the identity of hepatitis B infections, or to screen out blood donors carrying the virus.

4. Serological Tests

4.1 Assays for Hepatitis A Virus

A number of different tests are available in research laboratories. These include electron microscopy, complement fixation, immune adherence agglutination and solid phase radioimmunoassay. A new haemagglutination inhibition assay has been developed and is at present being clinically tested. Assays for use in routine hospital laboratories are likely to be developed within the next two or three years.

4.2 Assays for Hepatitis B virus

Serological methods available for detecting HBV infections are based on identification of antigen and/or antibodies associated with this infection. The tests are used primarily to establish the diagnosis of viral hepatitis B, to study its epidemiology, and to evaluate passive and active immunisation methods. The tests are also important to identify blood and plasma donors who are carriers of the disease.

A number of different techniques are available. These have differing sensitivity and their use is largely dictated by their complexity and cost. The most common screening procedure is the reverse passive haemagglutination assay and the most sensitive test is the radioimmunoassay.

Immunodiffusion Technique

This was the initial method used to detect HBsAg and, although insensitive and slow, it is also inexpensive, simple and specific. It is still used in some centres for screening purposes.

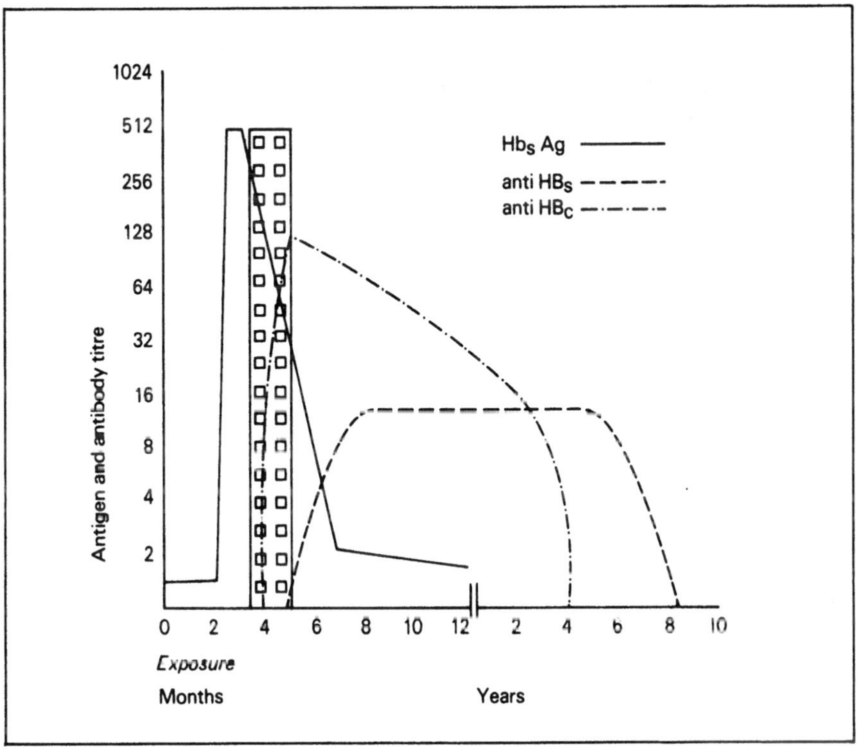

Fig. 1. The time course of a typical case of hepatitis B (from Crumpacker, 1976, with permission of the author).

Immunoelectrophoresis, Complement Fixation, and Reversed Passive Latex Agglutination

These techniques are up to ten times as sensitive as immunodiffusion and are used for detection of HBsAg. They are being used for screening purposes in some laboratories, but will give a considerable proportion of false positives (WHO Bulletin, 1977).

Radioimmunoassays

These are the most sensitive methods for detection of HBsAg and anti-HBs. Their high sensitivity and objectivity limit the number of false negative results. Their major disadvantage is their high cost.

Enzyme-linked Immunosorbent Assay (ELIZA)

This has been adapted for HBsAg detection and the technique shows a sensitivity similar to radioimmunoassay. Its acceptance for use will be dictated by cost and the availability of appropriate instrumentation.

Reverse Passive Haemagglutination

This method involves agglutination of erythrocytes coated with anti-HBs and is a sensitive method for detection of HBsAg. It is widely used for screening purposes. All the assays other than radioimmunoassay may give false negatives as they are less sensitive than the radio-label procedures.

5. Clinical Significance of HBV Antigens and Antibodies

Patients with acute hepatitis B may have detectable HBsAg in their blood for a period ranging from a few days to several months. The time lapse between exposure and appearance of the detectable serum HBsAg is related to the degree of infectivity of the inoculum. This time lapse may be as short as 2 to 3 weeks or as long as 3 or 4 months when the inoculum is low titre. Abnormal liver function tests and clinical symptoms appear some days or weeks after the initial appearance of HBsAg, often near the time when HBsAg levels are at their peak. In the majority of cases the disappearance of HBsAg and the subsequent appearance of anti-HBsAg signal recovery from HBV infection and the development of immunity to reinfection. In a small percentage, (5-10% of adults) the infection persists and HBsAg remains detectable for many months or years (fig. 1).

6. Summary of Laboratory and Immunological Findings

Leukocytopenia, lymphocytopenia and neutropenia may all be found in the preicteric phase. The serum bilirubin concentration is elevated and damage to the liver parenchyma results in increased activity of hepatocyte-derived enzymes, such as transaminases, in the blood. Hyperglobulinaemia and hypoalbuminaemia also occur. Bilirubin appears in the urine early, before the serum levels are elevated, and disappears while the serum level is still raised.

Detection of HBsAg or anti-HBsAg in a patient with clinical and laboratory evidence of hepatitis is considered diagnostic of hepatitis B infection.

References

Alter, H.J.; Purcell, R.H.; Holland, P.V. and Popper, H.: Transmissible agent in non-A, non-B hepatitis. Lancet 1: 461-463 (1978).

Crumpacker, C.S.: Hepatitis; in Remington and Klein (Eds) Infectious Diseases of the Fetus and Newborn Infant, p.492-520 (Saunders, Philadelphia 1976).

World Health Organisation: Advances in viral hepatitis. World Health Organisation Technical Report Series 602: 1-48 (1977).

Chapter VII

Toxoplasmosis

Toxoplasmosis is a disease resulting from infection by the protozoan parasite *Toxoplasma gondii*. *T. gondii* is found throughout the world and can infect most warm blooded animals. Most human populations show an incidence of past or present infection of between 20 and 50%, although figures as high as 95% have been recorded.

Toxoplasma has both sexual and asexual reproductive phases. The highly infectious oocyst is found only in the intestine of cats, while asexual cysts occur in tissues of many animals. Figure 1 shows schematically the sexual and asexual life cycle of *T. gondii*, modified from Hutchison's original description (Hutchison et al., 1970).

1. Mode of Infection

Cystic forms of toxoplasma are relatively heat resistant and can survive gastric juices. They have been found in skeletal muscle of sheep, swine and cattle. The sporulated oocysts are passed with cat faeces and become highly infectious within 24 to 48 hours by developing into sporocysts. These sporocysts are very resistant to adverse conditions and will survive in moist soils for months or even years.

Man can become infected by ingestion of poorly cooked meat that contains tissue cysts or by direct swallowing of oocysts from contaminated cat faeces. Direct transfer from man to man is unlikely but transplacental transfer from mother to fetus is a serious problem. Figure 2 illustrates the major routes of infection in man.

Parasitic proliferation at the site of entry allows dissemination via the lymphatics and the blood stream. Toxoplasma can develop in any type of host cell except the non-nucleated erythrocyte and can localise and multiply in any organ of the body, including the reticuloendothelial system, parenchymal cells of organs or the circulating system.

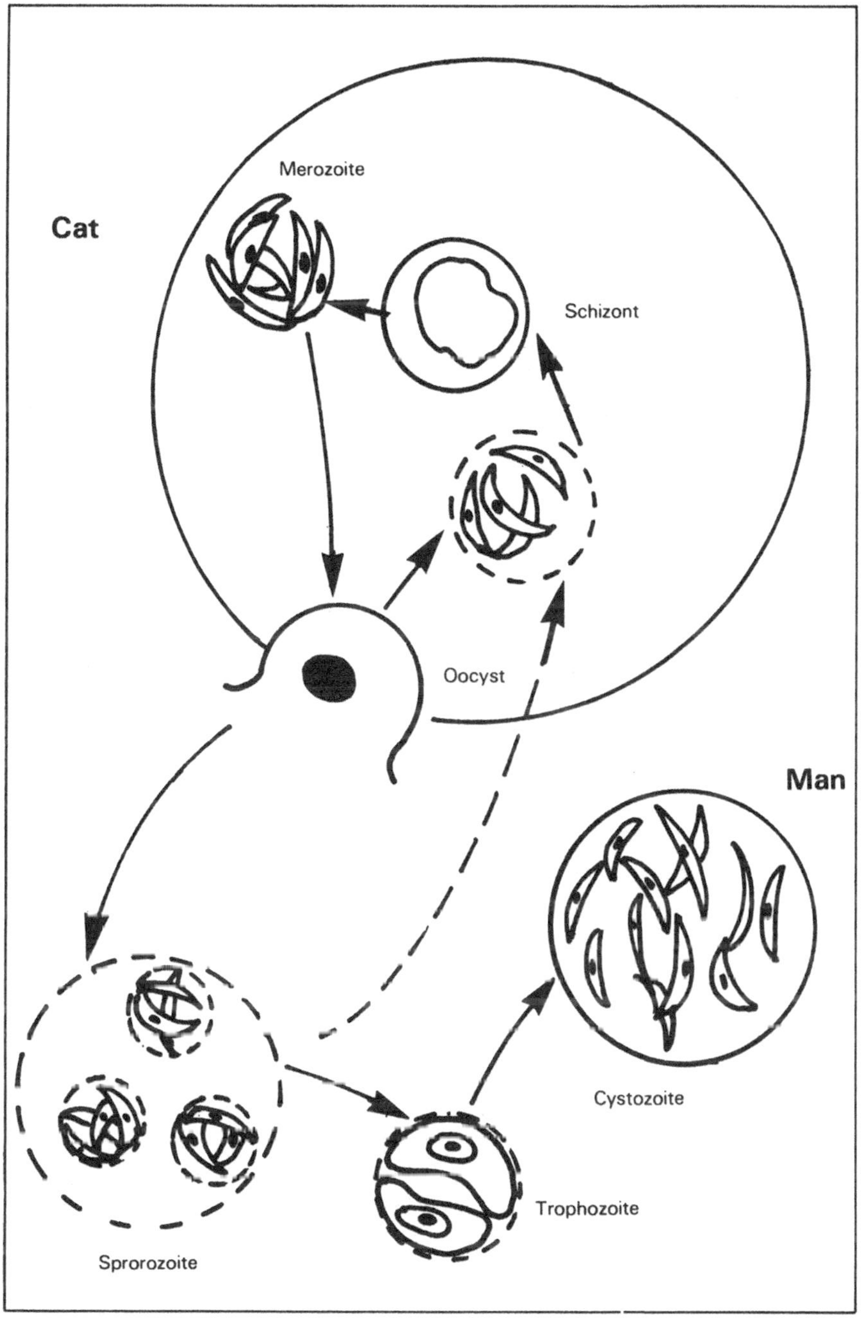

Fig. 1. The life cycle of *Toxoplasma gondii.*

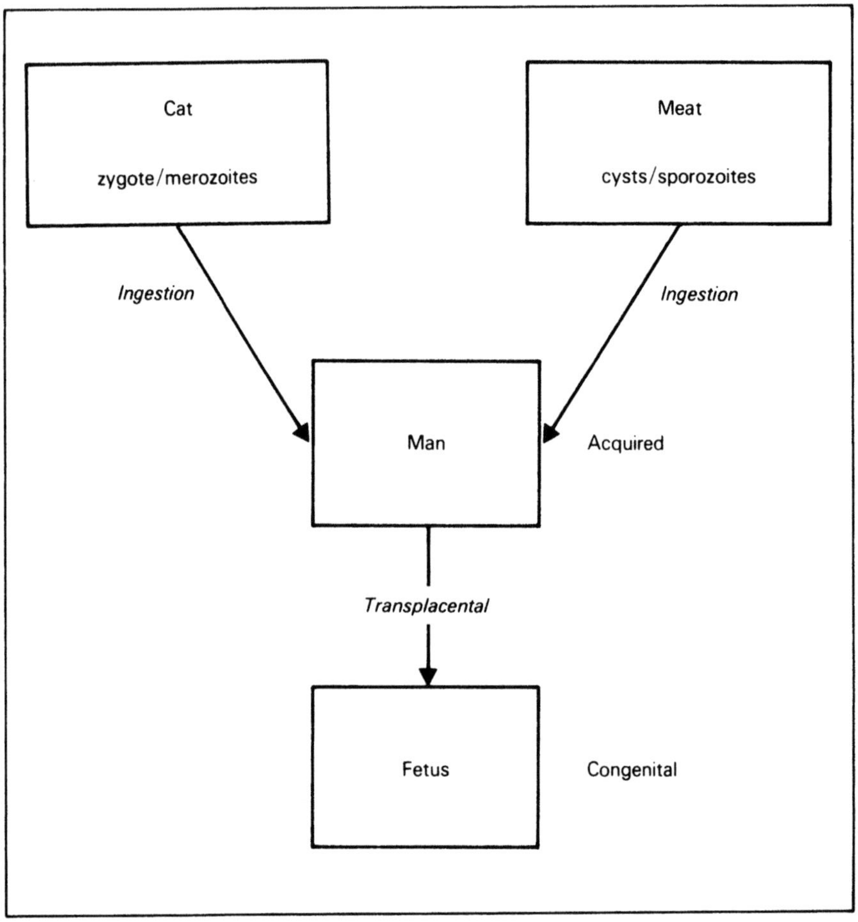

Fig. 2. The major routes of toxoplasma infection in man.

2. Disease Symptoms

Although infection in man is relatively common, clinically evident disease is rare. Clinical disease may be divided into two categories, acquired and congenital disease. Acquired toxoplasmosis may present in two ways, either as lymphadenopathy with or without involvement of other organs, or generalised toxoplasmosis. This may have symptoms similar to infectious mononucleosis, aseptic meningitis, hepatitis, myocarditis or pneumonitis. Malignancy, complement deficiencies and immunodeficiencies, and immunosuppressive therapy are among the predisposing factors which can affect the severity of the disease.

Congenital toxoplasmosis is the result of the mother having an active primary infection during pregnancy. The parasite crosses the placenta to infect the fetus. Risk

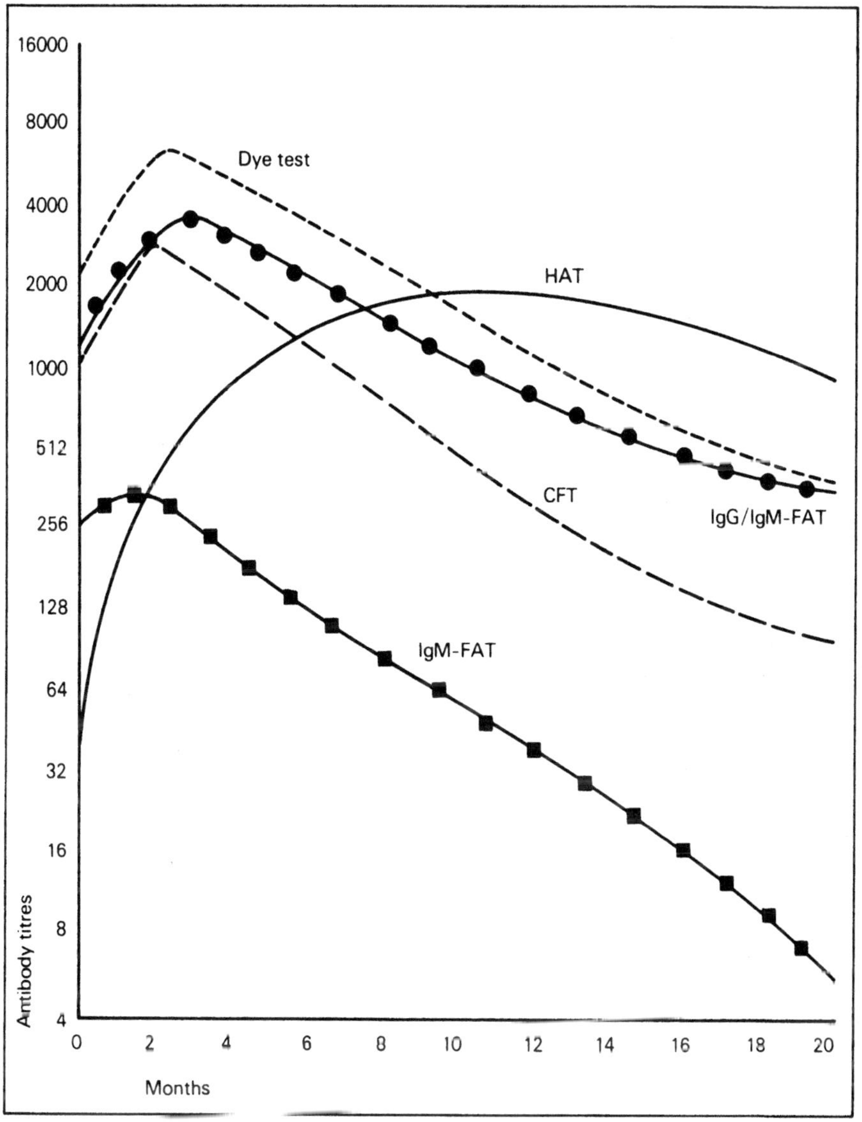

Fig. 3. Antibody curves in glandular toxoplasmosis (HAT = indirect haemagglutination test, FAT = fluorescent antibody test; CTF = complement fixation test). Adapted with permission of the authors from Karim and Ludlum (1975).

to the fetus is shown to be closely related to the time when maternal infection occurs. Infection of the mother during the first trimester results in a higher incidence of fetal infections but these are usually subclinical. Severe cases, at any stage of pregnancy, may result in abortion or severe congenital abnormalities. The eye is the most common site of congenital infection and the central nervous system can also be involved, producing a variety of symptoms.

Although congenital toxoplasmosis may be fatal, mothers of infected newborn are characteristically without symptoms. There is adequate evidence that other children born to mothers with inapparent infection, subsequent to the birth of a diseased child, will not be affected.

3. Antibodies to Toxoplasma

Toxoplasma organisms are antigenically very complex and consequently the antibodies produced are equally diverse. A characteristic pattern of antibody production is seen during the course of the disease. Soon after exposure to the parasite there is a rapid synthesis of IgM antibodies. These normally disappear during or shortly after the convalescent phase. At a later stage IgG antibodies are produced in high concentration. These are responsible for conferring immunity to the individual and can be found in the circulation for years. The IgG antibodies can be divided into 2 classes, complement-fixing and non-complement-fixing. The complement-fixing antibodies do not appear in the circulation as rapidly as those of the IgM class but do tend to disappear after adequate treatment, clinical improvement, or after the disease has subsided naturally. IgM antibodies are also capable of fixing complement and methods for detecting these antibodies are valuable in the diagnosis of active and recently acquired disease.

4. Laboratory Diagnosis

The diagnosis may be made in the laboratory by isolating the parasite, directly examining biopsied or necrotic material, or using immunological evidence.

4.1 Isolation

Definitive evidence of infection, by the isolation method, requires the use of susceptible animals, embryonated eggs or *in vitro* tissue culture cell lines. Emulsified material is most commonly inoculated into the brain or peritoneal cavity of young mice. Virulent toxoplasma will kill the mice within 3 to 6 weeks, but just prior to this stage the vegetative cystic form is found in large numbers in liver, spleen or peritoneum.

4.2 Direct Examination

Cystic or trophozoite forms may occasionally be observed by microscopic analysis of tissue or body fluids with Romanowsky stains. However, because numbers of parasites are very sparse such a procedure is rarely successful.

The direct examination of infected material by fluorescent labelled anti-toxoplasma serum is a highly sensitive and reliably specific test for detection of toxoplasma antigenic material in placental, fetal and lymph tissue. Such material can be misdiagnosed by conventional histology.

4.3 Immunological Tests

Immunological tests for assaying specific toxoplasma antibodies still dominate laboratory diagnosis. Numerous tests have been devised of which 4 have been demonstrated to have the most value. These are the dye exclusion test, the complement fixation test, the indirect haemagglutination test and the fluorescent antibody test.

Dye Exclusion Test (DT)

Although the DT is probably still the most specific and sensitive of these tests few laboratories undertake this procedure routinely because of inherent difficulties in standardisation and the necessity for continual maintenance of the toxoplasma strains.

The DT was developed by Sabin and Feldman and these workers found that staining of living toxoplasma with basic methylene blue is inhibited after the organisms have been incubated with specific antiserum and fresh human serum (Sabin and Feldman, 1948). When an unknown serum is examined the dilution is determined which prevents staining of 50% of the toxoplasma counted.

The DT detects both acute and latent phases of the disease. Titres of at least 1 : 1000 seem to indicate acute toxoplasmosis, especially when associated with titres of 1 : 10 or more in the complement fixation test (see below).

Complement Fixation Test (CFT)

The CFT uses an extract produced from chorioallantoic membranes of infected chicken eggs as an antigen. It is freed from all solid particles by high speed centrifugation. To exclude nonspecific reactions an extract from non-infected chorioallantoic membranes is used as a control.

The rise of complement-fixing antibodies in an infestation begins later than those antibodies shown by the DT. The titres reach a much lower peak value and fall below the level of identification within weeks and months. Positive values with the CFT, especially in connection with high titres in the dye test, indicate an active disease process.

Haemagglutination Test (HAT)

This test is sensitive and specific. It requires an antigen prepared from pure suspensions of parasites which must be stored in the frozen or lyophilised state. In general, good qualitative agreement has been found between the HAT test and the DT but the former requires standardisation in each individual laboratory.

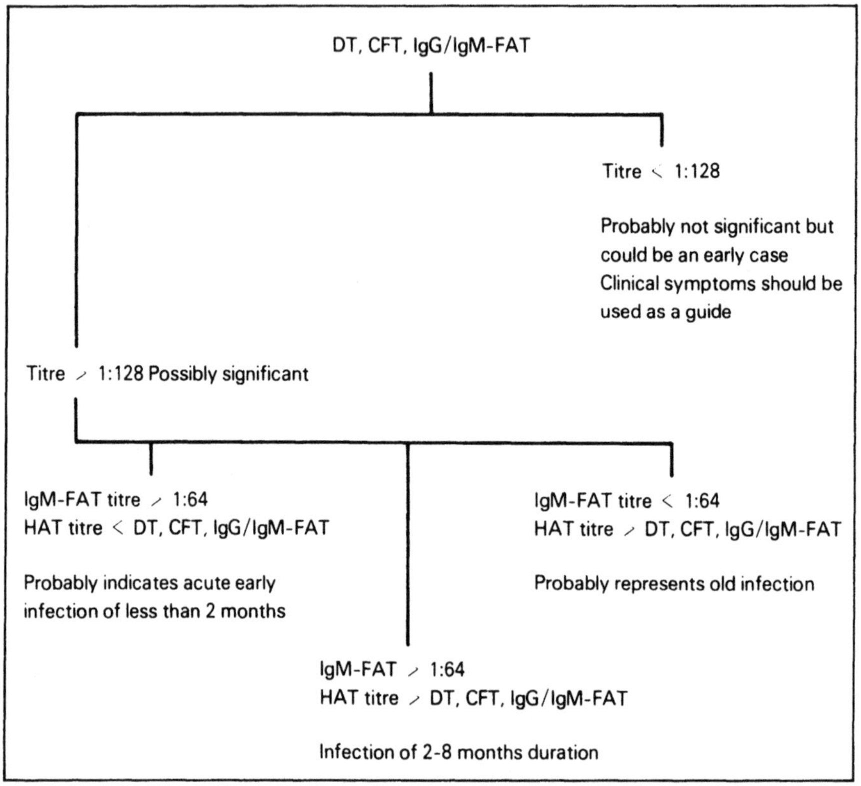

Fig. 4. Different serological tests using a single sample may be utilised to determine the stage of toxoplasma infection (see fig. 3 for key). Adapted with permission of the authors from Karim and Ludlum (1975).

HAT titres become positive and rise more slowly than DT titres and unless increased sensitivity is achieved the test cannot be used as the only test in suspected cases of active congenital or acquired toxoplasmosis. Its use at present is in the diagnosis of chronic infections, such as ocular toxoplasmosis, and the HAT test supplements the DT in the diagnosis of acute disease because of the slower rise of HAT antibodies. It has been used successfully in sero-epidemiological studies.

Fluorescent Antibody Test (FAT)

This test utilises killed and lyophilised toxoplasma. This is fixed to a slide and antibodies are detected by an indirect immunofluorescence procedure whereby a patient's serum is added to the slide and, after washing, anti-toxoplasma antibodies are visualised with fluorescein-labelled anti-human antibody under UV light. Positive preparations are easily recognised by a fluorescent edge to the organism. A better contrast can be obtained if Evan's blue is added to the conjugated anti-human globulin because this gives a red fluorescence.

This technique is proving increasingly useful because it produces titres which correspond to the values of the DT, but it has the advantage of being a much simpler method of examination; in many laboratories it has replaced the DT as a diagnostic method. It is additionally useful in that with the use of a suitable antisera, the immunoglobulin class of the antibody can be established and thus conclusions drawn in regard to the stage of the infection.

The detection of IgM antibodies by the FAT is regarded as the method of choice in the identification of toxoplasmosis of the newborn. IgG antibodies can pass the placental barrier but IgM antibodies cannot and thus the finding of IgM antibodies in the newborn suggests neonatal infection.

4.4 Evaluation of Test Methods

Immunological tests, while not diagnostic for toxoplasmosis, almost exclude active disease when a negative result is obtained. A satisfactory serological diagnosis of toxoplasmosis should be based on the demonstration of a 4-fold or more change in antibody titre. Figure 3 shows that the majority of antibodies have reached high levels after about 8 weeks and that these high titres may persist for months or years. Because sera are often not obtained very early in the disease, maximum use must be made of a single serum sample if repeated tests show static antibody levels (fig. 4). The HAT curve differs from those of the CFT, DT and IgG/IgM FAT. The latter three follow parallel courses and seem to measure the same antibody. The IgM/FAT differs from the others in that it is specific in measuring only IgM antibodies.

The DT remains probably the most specific and sensitive of the tests discussed. However, the difficulties associated with this test mean that few laboratories use it as a routine test. The standard assay used by most laboratories is the FAT.

References

Hutchison, W.M.; Dunrachie, J.F.; Sim, N.C. and Work, K.: Coccidian-like nature of *Toxoplasma gondii*. British Medical Journal 1: 142-144 (1970).

Karim, K.A. and Ludlum, G.B.: The relationship and significance of antibody titres as determined by various serological methods in glandular and ocular toxoplasmosis. Journal of Clinical Pathology 28: 42-49 (1975).

Sabin, A.B. and Feldman, H.A.: Dyes as microchemical indicators of a new immunity phenomenon affecting a protozoan parasite (toxoplasma). Science 108: 660-662 (1948)

Further Reading

World Health Organisation: Toxoplasmosis. Report of WHO Meeting of Investigators. Technical Report Series 431: 1-31 (1969).

Chapter VIII

Hydatids

Hydatid disease is caused by the larval stages of the canine tapeworm *Echinococcus granulosus*. Echinococcus has a worldwide distribution with most frequent infestation occurring in areas of concentrated sheep and cattle husbandry; figure 1 illustrates its life-cycle. Because it presents with few specific clinical symptoms or signs a good deal of reliance has been placed upon the various immunological tests which are available to aid in the diagnosis of hydatid disease.

1. Clinical Features

Two patterns of symptoms occur: firstly, and most commonly, patients present with signs of a space-occupying lesion. On occasion multiple cysts can be present. Clinical details are nonspecific and relative to the site of growth of the cyst. Secondly, occasionally cysts rupture and the patient, being presented with a massive load of foreign protein, may experience an anaphylactic reaction which can be fatal.

2. Diagnosis

In some patients, whose cysts are calcified, the diagnosis can be made by x-ray. Eosinophilia offers suggestive evidence but serological tests are the prime diagnostic aid. The correct diagnosis is necessary before surgical intervention. Immunological tests are used to monitor the patient's postoperative state and to determine the degree of success of the surgery.

Specific antibodies are found in the blood of hydatid patients and these are used as the basis for immunological tests. Continuous access to the antigenic substances produced by the parasite can result in a state of hypersensitivity in the patient. The cysts which are found in the liver usually contain the greatest amount of antigenic substance.

The allergic syndrome may be caused by an intradermal diagnostic test or by accidental or spontaneous rupture of a cyst. The intensity of the reaction is governed by the hypersensitivity of the patient and the amount of antigenic fluid which enters the blood. Two differing immunological protocols have been used for diagnosis since the early 1900's with variable success, namely intradermal testing and measurement of specific humoral antibodies.

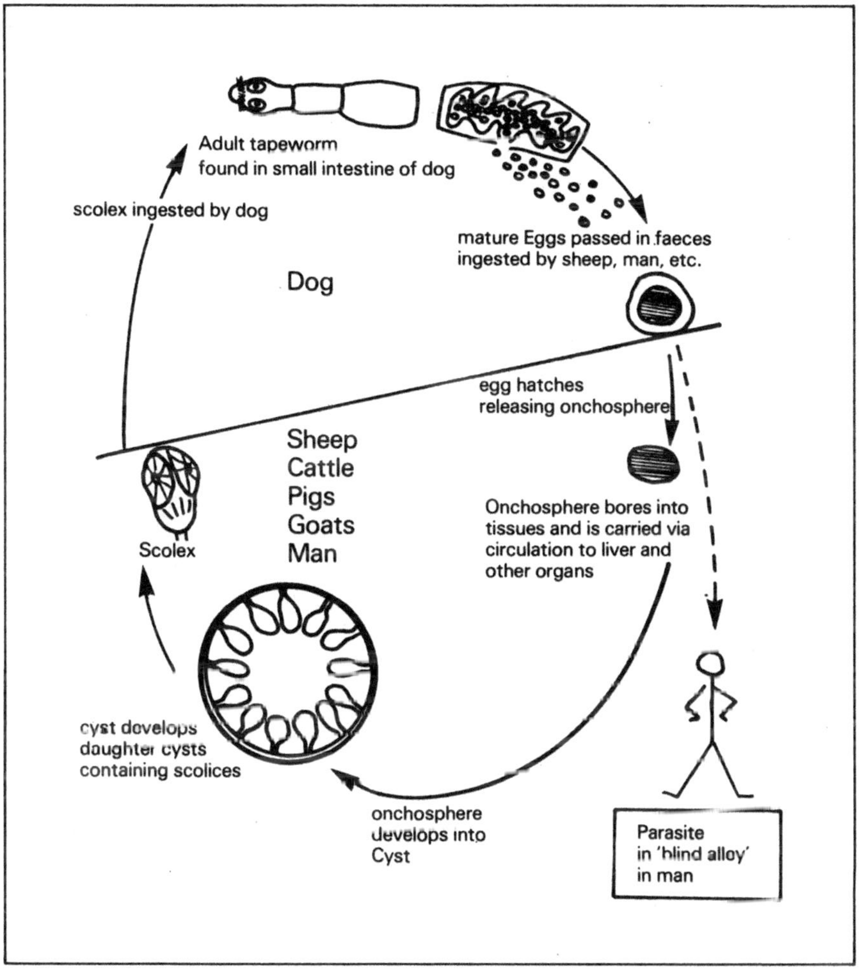

Fig. 1. The life cycle of *Echinococcus granulosa.*

Table I. Comparative efficacy of diagnostic tests for hydatids, according to the type of infection

Test	Percentage positive			False positive %
	Hepatic	Pulmonary	Recurrent	
Haemagglutination	90	65	100	< 2
Complement fixation	80	60	95	< 5
Fluorescent test	96	60	100	12-15
Latex particles	80	55	95	10-15
Casoni intradermal	85	60	90	15-20

2.1 Intradermal Testing — the Casoni Test

The basis of the Casoni test is the injection of human or animal hydatid fluid into the dermis of the patient. The Casoni test gives both an immediate reaction, which appears after about 15 minutes, and a delayed phase which develops after 24 hours (Kagan et al., 1966). The immediate response is generally considered to be more sensitive but less specific for the diagnosis of hydatid disease. In the immediate phase an urticarial papule, indicating a positive result, is seen in nearly 90% of hydatid cases but there can be up to 15% false positive readings caused by such conditions as carcinomatosis, leishmaniasis and taeniasis.

The delayed response offers better discrimination but the test is reactive in less than 70% of patients with active disease. As previously mentioned the allergic nature of hydatid disease is well recognised and anaphylactic shock in sensitised patients can result, not only from rupture of the cyst, but also through repeated Casoni testing.

A further disadvantage of the Casoni test is that positive results persist for many years after successful removal of the hydatid cyst and this makes the test useless for assistance in postoperative follow-up.

2.2 Tests for Specific Humoral Antibodies

The most commonly used tests are complement fixation, haemagglutination, latex agglutination, fluorescent antibody and crossed electrophoresis techniques.

Complement Fixation (CF)

The complement fixation test, which is similar to the Wasserman reaction has been utilised for many years but has suffered from lack of both sensitivity and apparent specificity. The sensitivity can be significantly enhanced if careful standardisation of hydatid antigen is carried out to ensure optimum dilution. This procedure reduces the incidence of nonspecific reactions which are caused by minor antigens which cross react with other helminths. CF antibodies when detected are of diagnostic and prognostic importance, as their presence generally denotes current or recent infection and therefore acts as a reliable indicator of disease activity. CF antibodies revert to negative within a year of successful surgery (Lass et al., 1973).

Haemagglutination (HA)

The haemagglutination test utilises stabilised red blood cells which have been tagged with hydatid antigen. It is a highly sensitive test (90-95% positive with live hydatids) and is also remarkably specific, for few false positive reactions (titres $> 1:400$) occur even in healthy individuals residing in areas where hydatids are endemic. High HA levels may persist for years after successful surgery.

Immunofluorescence and Latex Agglutination Tests (FAT, LA)

The fluorescent antibody test and the latex agglutination test both demonstrate adequate sensitivity but both exhibit a high incidence of false positive reactions. Between 12 and 50% of individuals with hepatic diseases other than hydatids have demonstrated positive FA and positive latex agglutination tests at low titre (Kagan et al., 1960).

Simultaneous use of HA and CF tests will allow for a higher incidence of true positive results and also gives the best prognostic indications (table I). At present there seems little advantage in using FA or latex tests for the diagnosis of hydatids.

References

Kagan, I.G.; Norman, L.; Allain, D.S. and Goodchild C.G.: Studies on echinococcosis: nonspecific serological reaction of hydatid fluid antigen with serum of patients ill with diseases other than echinococcosis. Journal of Immunology 84: 635-640 (1960).

Kagan, I.G.; Oximan, J.J.; Varela, J.C. and Allain, D.S.: Evaluation of intradermal and serologic tests for the diagnosis of hydatid disease. Journal of Tropical Medicine 15: 172-181 (1966).

Lass, N.; Laver, Z. and Lengy, J.: The immunodiagnosis of hydatid disease: post-operative evaluation of the skin test and four serological tests. Annals of Allergy 31: 430-436 (1973).

Further Reading

Lewis, J.W., Jr.; Koss, N. and Kerstein, M.D.: A review of echinococcus disease. Annals of Surgery 181: 390-396 (1975).

Little, J.M.: Hydatid disease at Royal Prince Alfred Hospital 1964-1974. Medical Journal of Australia 1: 903-908 (1976).

Chapter IX

Syphilis

Syphilis is a venereal disease caused by the spirochaete micro-organism *Treponema pallidum*. As this organism cannot be cultured on artificial media the diagnosis of syphilis depends on the correlation of clinical data with additional information provided by serological tests.

Recent changes in the immunological procedures for diagnosing syphilis, particularly the adoption of the specific treponemal tests, have rationalised the subject and simplified the interpretation of results.

1. Clinical Features

Although the disease is a continuum, clinical and laboratory evaluation is assisted by considering the disease as having different stages. Early syphilis includes primary and secondary stages and late syphilis is referred to as tertiary syphilis (fig. 1).

1.1 Primary Syphilis

After an incubation period of between 9 and 90 days (average 3 weeks) primary syphilis may be recognised by the appearance of a chancre, usually at the site of inoculation.

1.2 Secondary Syphilis

About two months after exposure, symptoms of secondary syphilis appear. These include flu-like symptoms, skin eruptions and general lymphadenopathy.

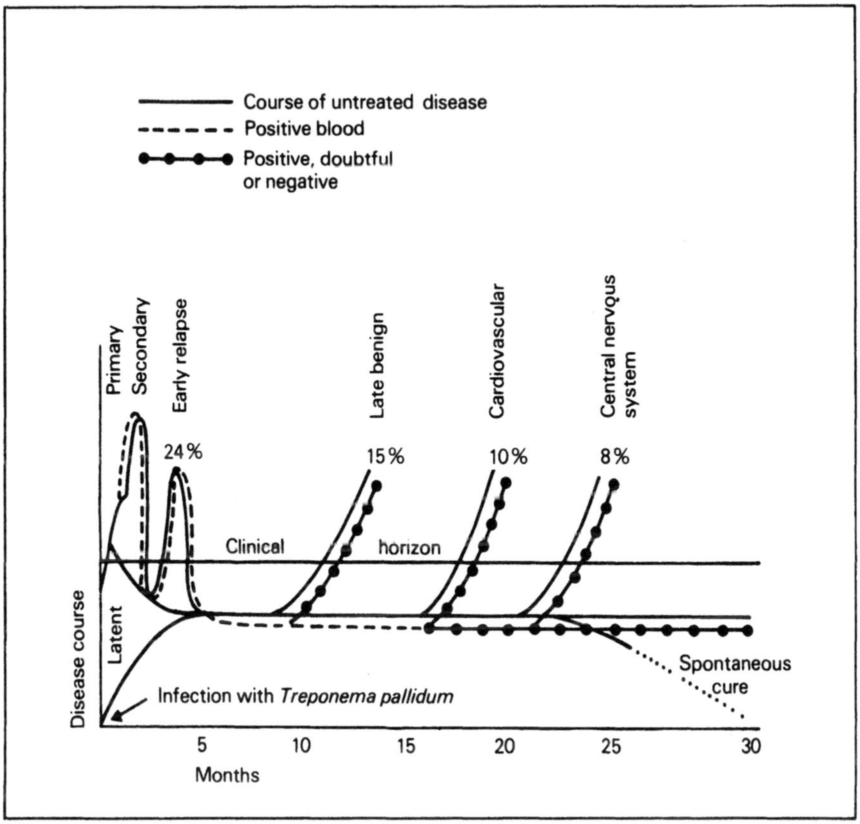

Fig. 1. Disease course of untreated, acquired syphilis. From Kampmieir (1964) with permission of the author.

1.3 Latent Syphilis

Latent syphilis is characterised by repeated positive serological tests for syphilis with an absence of any symptoms or clinical features of the disease. The term early latent syphilis usually refers to infections of less than four years' duration.

1.4 Tertiary Syphilis

In untreated patients the symptoms of late syphilis may appear anywhere between 2 and 10 years after the initial infection. Inflammation occurs, either gummatous and localised, or chronic and diffuse. Gummas may develop anywhere in the body but they are found most frequently on the skin, in bones or the upper respiratory tract. There may be involvement of the cardiovascular system (cardiovascular syphilis) and neurosyphilis develops in approximately 10% of untreated cases.

Demonstration of sequential changes in antibody levels is often useful in determining the stage of syphilis or whether treatment has been successful.

1.5 Congenital Syphilis

A pregnant woman with syphilis can transfer the infection via the placenta to the developing fetus.

2. Immunology of Syphilis

It is not clear whether man has a significant natural immunity to syphilis. The main defence mechanisms against infection appear to be maintenance of intact skin and mucous membrane barriers.

Treponemal species are widespread in nature and many animals harbour a treponemal flora. Antigenic components from these commensal organisms (which are also common to virulent *T. pallidum)* may confer low grade immunity in man. Observations in areas where treponemal diseases such as yaws and pinta are prevalent show that there is little venereal disease, and this suggests that adults in these areas are protected against *T. pallidum* as a result of childhood infection with other treponemas. Conversely, in areas where yaws and pinta have been eradicated, endemic venereal syphilis is now seen. There is no complete immunity to syphilis because reinfection may occur, despite the prior presence of treponemal antibodies. Resistance to reinfection does increase according to the length of time the initial infection has been left untreated. Very early in infection serum antibody activity is confined primarily to the macroglobulin class (IgM) and this is rapidly overtaken by the 7S antibody (IgG). Very late in the infection, and after adequate treatment, the only reactivity observed is in the IgG fraction.

Multiple antibodies are produced during treponemal infection (table I) and these can be divided into 3 groups:

i) *Reagin or non-treponemal antibodies*
These appear as a consequence of syphilis and many other diseases. They cross react with a number of antigens from other tissues, e.g. extracts of heart muscle.

ii) *Group treponemal antibodies*
These are directed against somatic antigens which are common to all treponemes.

iii) *Specific treponemal antibodies*
These are directed against antigens specific for *T. pallidum*. Because these antibodies appear at different times during the various clinical stages of the

Table 1. Humoral antibodies characteristic of syphilis and their relationship to serological tests for syphilis. From Johnson (1972) with permission of the author

Antibodies	Antigen	Tests
Reagin, nonspecific antibodies that appear as a consequence of syphilis and many other diseases	Lipid extracts of normal human and non-human tissues suffice; cardiolipin as now in use is a highly purified lipid extract of beef heart combined with lecithin and cholesterol	Complement fixation: Wassermann Kolmer Flocculation: VDRL (Venereal Disease Research Laboratory) Kahn
Specifically antitreponemal	*Treponema pallidum* Reiter strain (avirulent)	RPCF (Reiter protein complement fixation) TPI (*Treponema pallidum* immunobilisation)
	Nichols strain (virulent)	FTA (fluorescent treponemal antibody) FTA-ABS (fluorescent treponemal antibody absorption)

disease several tests should be performed simultaneously to give a conclusive result.

3. Diagnosis of Syphilis

The diagnosis is suggested by the patient's history and the finding of skin lesions of primary or secondary syphilis or clinical features compatible with tertiary disease. At some stages organisms can be detected in infected lesions but the diagnosis depends principally on the serological tests.

3.1 Reagin or Non-treponemal Tests

There are two types of test — flocculation and complement fixation. The Venereal Disease Research Laboratory (VDRL) and Rapid Plasma Reagin (RPR) are slide tests of the flocculation type and the Wasserman reaction (WR) is the most common complement fixation procedure. These tests utilise cardiolipin/lecithin extracts from normal mammalian tissue as an antigen source. They play an important role in

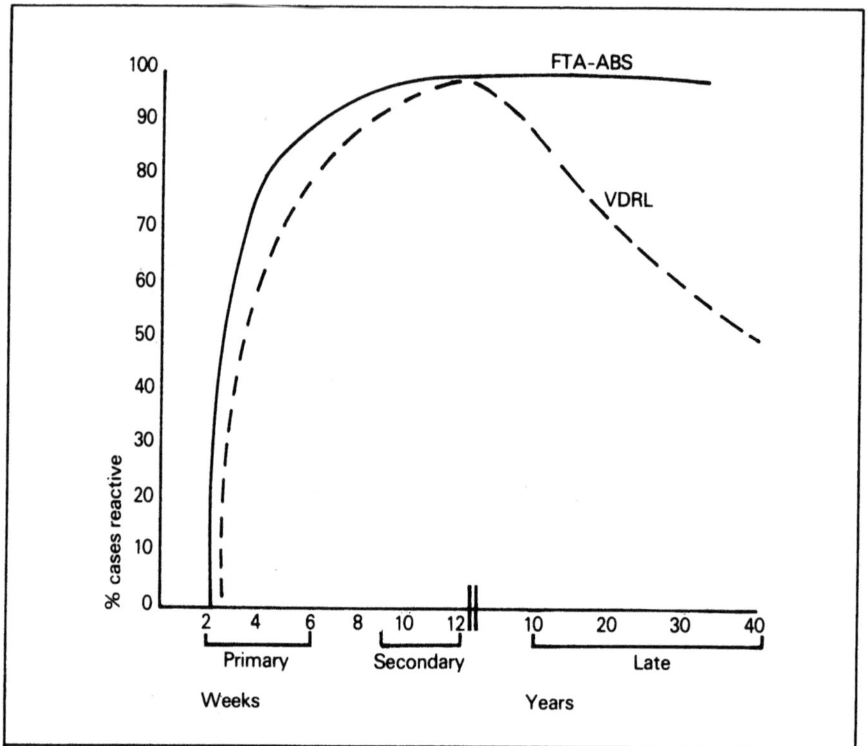
FTA-ABS
VDRL
% cases reactive
100
90
80
70
60
50
40
30
20
10
0
2
4
6
8
10
12
10
20
30
40
Primary
Secondary
Late
Weeks
Years

2

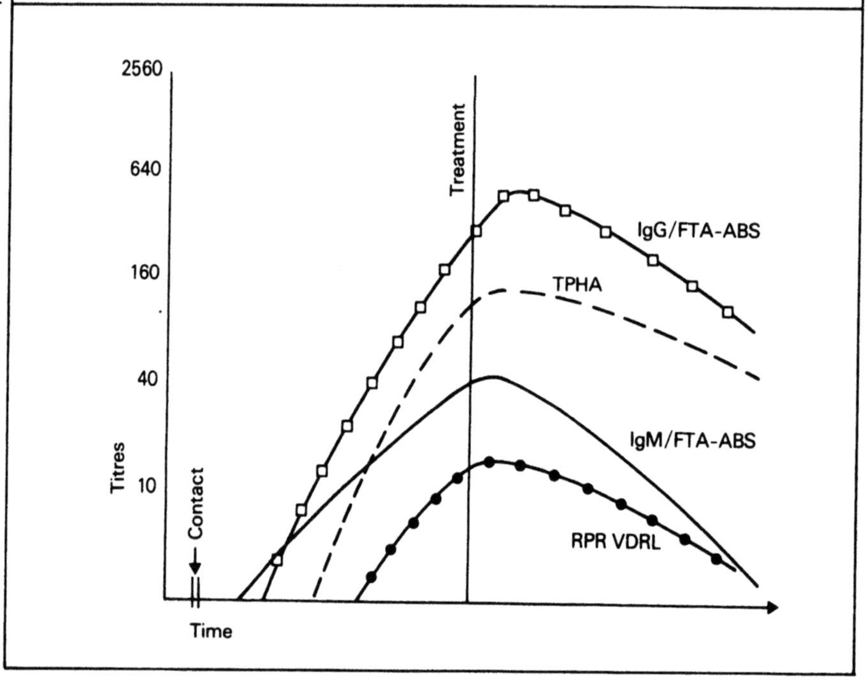
Treatment
IgG/FTA-ABS
TPHA
IgM/FTA-ABS
RPR VDRL
Titres
2560
640
160
40
10
Contact
Time

3

the diagnosis of syphilis because they are simple, can be quantitated and are ideally suited for screening large batteries of sera at one time. These tests remain the standard for screening purposes and monitoring the immunological response to treatment. A quantitative response is informative because reagin antibody levels generally fall off quite quickly after adequate chemotherapy.

Because reagin antibody response is usually not detected until 3 to 5 weeks after exposure, tests are often of either low titre or negative in early primary syphilis but high levels ($\geqslant 1:32$) are often observed in secondary syphilis with variable levels detected in later stages (figs. 2 & 3).

Because the lipoidal antigens are extracted from normal mammalian tissue falsely reactive tests are sometimes observed (section 3.6).

3.2 Group Treponemal Tests

The Reiter Complement Fixation Test (RCFT) is a relatively simple procedure for detecting this type of antibody. The antigen used is a protein extract obtained from a saprophytic strain of treponema *(T. reiteri)* grown on an artificial medium. This method has fallen into disfavour because it is insensitive in both early primary and late syphilis and therefore has limited use. False reactions may also occur because of nonspecific interactions with a lipopolysaccharide impurity in the antigen material.

3.3 Specific Treponemal Tests

T. Pallidum Immobilisation Test (TPI)

The first specific treponemal test was described in 1949 by Nelson and Mayer and was called the *T. pallidum* immobilisation (TPI) test (Nelson and Mayer, 1949). This method demonstrates the ability of a specific antibody in the presence of complement to immobilise living *T. pallidum* micro-organisms. Because these immobilising antibodies develop slowly, 60% of patients with primary syphilis and 30% with secondary syphilis may have negative TPI tests. As the test lacks sensitivity, needs a high degree of technical skill to perform and is difficult to standardise, further methods were sought to simplify diagnosis.

Fig. 2. Serology of untreated syphilis (FTA/ABS = fluorescent treponemal antibody absorption test; VDRL = Venereal Disease Research Laboratory test). Adapted from Pusch (1974) with permission of author and editors.

Fig. 3. Serology of treated syphilis (see text for detail of tests).

Table II. A comparison of reactivity to immunological tests at varying stages of syphilis (see text for details of tests)

Disease state	Percentage positive			
	FTA-ABS	TPHA	TPI	RPR
Primary syphilis	90	85	60	80
Secondary syphilis	95-100	95-100	85	95-100
Late syphilis	95-100	95-100	90-95	80
Latent syphilis	95-100	95-100	90-95	80

Fluorescent Treponemal Antibody Absorption Test (FTA-ABS)

The FTA-ABS test detects specific treponemal antibodies slightly earlier in the infection than the TPHA test (see below). Extensive research has revealed that the FTA-ABS test is capable of detecting 85 to 90% of patients with primary syphilis and 95 to 100% of those with all other forms (Hunter, 1975). With the good monospecific antiglobulin reagents available commercially a specific IgM FTA-ABS test can now be performed to which most patients with early primary syphilis will be reactive.

Because it is both sensitive and specific the FTA-ABS procedure has now replaced the TPI and RCFT in most reference laboratories and has become the method of choice for diagnosing syphilis.

T. Pallidum Haemagglutination Test (TPHA)

The TPHA appears to detect mainly IgG antibodies and becomes reactive at about the same time as the IgG FTA-ABS. The TPHA does not require expensive microscopic equipment or a high degree of technical skill and therefore it may be used to test large batteries of test samples (McKay, 1972). This 'micro' haemagglutination method is very suitable for screening purposes because it can detect at least 95% of all stages of syphilis except very early primary disease.

Table II lists the comparative efficacy of the immunological tests described.

3.4 Identification of Syphilis in Lesion Material

Using dark ground microscopy a diagnosis of syphilis can be made by demonstrating *T. pallidum* in the lesions found in the early stages of the disease. In late skin lesions or gummas it is difficult because the number of treponemes is very small. Problems in identification of pathogenic organisms are increased because there are normally saprophytic spirochaetes found in oral and genital lesions. A negative result does not necessarily mean that the patient does not have syphilis and false negative results can be caused by a number of factors:

1) The patient may have received prior treatment
2) The lesion may be healing
3) The lesion may be from a patient with late syphilis.

Despite these drawbacks a positive dark ground test, particularly in early primary syphilis, allows a diagnosis and the patient can receive prompt treatment before detectable antigens have developed.

Preparations from genital lesions with insufficient treponemes and oral lesions which contain commensal flora such as *T. microdentium* have made interpretation of conventional dark ground microscopy difficult. Fluorescent antibody techniques have now been developed which can be used with confidence to identify *T. pallidum* from exudate material from both early and late stages of disease.

A reagent can be used for direct and indirect immunofluorescent procedures which enables specimens to be collected into capillary tubes, or onto slides as a thin film, without the need to have laboratory facilities in close proximity.

3.5 Identification of Congenital Syphilis

The diagnosis of congenital syphilis can be made on clinical grounds alone if the infant presents with typical clinical signs and a positive dark ground lesion. However diagnosis is difficult when the neonate presents without symptoms but is seroreactive.

The IgM FTA-ABS test was developed to distinguish between syphilitic babies and those with reactive tests resulting from passive transplacental passage of maternal IgG antibody. As IgM antibody is too large to pass across the placental barrier, the presence of IgM treponemal antibodies in umbilical cord or fetal serum is now considered as definite evidence of active congenital infection, as long as placental leakage during delivery has been excluded (O'Neill, 1976).

A negative IgM FTA-ABS performed at birth does not exclude congenital syphilis as some neonates will not produce IgM treponemal antibodies until they are 3 months old. Conversely, passively transferred IgG antibody will disappear from the baby's blood within 3 months; therefore persistently high titre IgG FTA-ABS reaction for longer than 3 months can also be taken as evidencc of intrauterine syphilis infection.

3.6 False Positive Reactions

False positive reactions will occur with both reaginic and specific treponemal assays; the former are also referred to as biological false positives and may have serious implications.

Table III. Conditions associated with biological false positive (BFP) reactions to reaginic serologic tests for syphilis

Acute BFP (less than 6 months)	Systemic sclerosis
Infectious mononucleosis	Rheumatoid arthritis
Infectious hepatitis	Sjogren's syndrome
Measles	
Chicken pox	Discoid lupus
Viral pneumonia	Hashimoto's thyroiditis
Upper respiratory tract infections	Cirrhosis of liver
Recent vaccinations	Heroin addiction
	Malaria
Chronic BFP (longer than 6 months)	Leprosy
Systemic lupus erythematosus	Tuberculosis
Polyarteritis	Leptospirosis

A problem not easily solved is the appearance of a false positive FTA-ABS test which has been observed in pregnant patients or those with systemic lupus erythematosus (SLE). In SLE an atypical 'beaded' fluorescent pattern is due to the complexing of anti-DNA and DNA from the treponema nucleus which has been extruded through breaks in the micro-organism's cell wall. In normal pregnancy false reactions with FTA-ABS reactions are fortunately rare and when they do occur, tend to be transient. Sera with high titre rheumatoid factor antibodies may also non-specifically react in the FTA-ABS test and give a false positive IgM FTA-ABS test. This problem is difficult to solve and it may need several absorptions of the test sera with aggregated gammaglobulin before all rheumatoid factor is removed (Hunter, 1975).

A *biological* false positive reaction may be defined as a positive reaction with one or more of the reagin tests in the absence of a history or clinical evidence of syphilis, and with negative specific tests of antibodies to *T. pallidum* (table III). Lipoidal antigens used in reagin tests are found in many normal tissues; therefore it is not surprising that these tests are sometimes falsely positive.

There are two types of biological false positive reaction — acute and chronic. The acute type generally develops during or shortly after an acute infection, or as a primary response to vaccination. Recognised causes of acute biological false reactions are pregnancy, malaria and upper respiratory tract infection. The chronic type is persistently reactive, i.e. a reaction lasts for more than 6 months. There are 3 groups of patients who show these chronic false positive reactions:

1) Those with no clinical disease
2) Those with a disease known to produce a chronic reaction
3) Those who suffer from arthritis, fever or malaise.

Up to 40% of chronic false positive tests for syphilis are observed in SLE or related connective tissue diseases as well as diseases such as brucellosis, pernicious

Table IV. Interpretation of reaction patterns to the various immunological tests for syphilis

Test				Interpretation
WR/RPR	TPHA	FA/ABS		
		IgM	IgG.	
±	–	+	–	Early primary syphilis
+	+	±	+	Undetected primary and latent syphilis
±	+	–	+	Treated syphilis, or yaws
–	±	–	+	Treated primary syphilis
+	–	–	–	Biological false positive (BFP)

anaemia, lymphatic leukaemia and metastatic cancer. Chronic biological false positive reactions are often useful in identifying immune deficiency.

True biological false positive reactions will invariably have a negative TPHA or FTA-ABS so a distinction between syphilis and false reaction can be reliably made.

As pathogenic treponemas of syphilis, yaws, pinta and bejel are antigenically very similar, there are no immunological tests capable of differentiating these diseases. This presents great problems when trying to distinguish normal seropositive people, from areas where yaws and pinta were once endemic, from those patients who currently have venereal disease. The IgM FTA-ABS test can be helpful in these cases.

3.7 Current Status of IgM Treponemal Tests

It is necessary to identify patients with active venereal disease. Recent evidence convincingly demonstrates that IgM antibodies occur before other immunoglobulins in most infectious diseases. Individuals who have been infected with yaws during childhood are usually reactive to treponemal antigens for life. In such cases the IgM FTA-ABS is extremely useful, for if reactive it is indicative of recently acquired syphilis. As already stated patients previously cured of syphilis are not necessarily immune, so that the appearance of IgM treponemal antibodies warns the physician that reinfection may have occurred. This information is valuable in assessing early reinfections in homosexual populations as up to 20% may have had a previous syphilitic infection.

In early primary syphilis IgM treponemal antibodies will predominate. Such antibodies are of prime importance at a time when reagin antibodies and IgG treponemal antibodies cannot be demonstrated. The usefulness of the IgM FTA-ABS in congenital syphilis has been considered separately above.

Summary

Table IV shows in simplified form the rationale of reaction patterns that can be obtained by using the various immunological tests for syphilis. Regardless of the patterns obtained, three basic facts should be considered when interpreting the results, and table IV highlights these points:

1) Detection of treponemal antibodies with tests such as FTA-ABS or TPHA is necessary for the diagnosis of early syphilis
2) IgM and later IgG antibodies are present in *active* untreated infection
3) IgM antibodies tend to disappear after the infection has been adequately treated, but IgG antibodies remain.

Because IgM treponemal antibodies may not always disappear completely with treatment, detecting reagin antibody levels is a more reliable method when assessing antibiotic therapy. Specific treponemal tests as well as reagin tests should always be performed in parallel if one is to exclude venereal syphilis, while the IgM FTA-ABS should be performed where reaction patterns are difficult to interpret and supporting clinical history is inconclusive.

References

Catterall, R.D.: Systemic disease and the biological false positive reaction. British Journal of Venereal Disease 48: 1-12 (1972).

Hunter, E.F.: The fluorescent treponemal antibody-absorption (FTA-Abs) test for syphilis. Critical Reviews in Clinical Laboratory Science 5: 315-353 (1975).

Johnson, T.W.: Syphilis: in Hoeprich (Ed) Infectious Diseases p.543-552 (Harper and Row, New York 1972).

Kampmieir, R.H.: The late manifestations of syphilis. Medical Clinics of North America 48: 669-697 (1964).

McKay, E.J.: Micro TPHA-comparison with other serological tests for syphilis. New Zealand Journal of Medical Laboratory Technology 26: 102-106 (1972).

Nelson, R. and Mayer, M.M.: Immobilization of Treponema pallidum in vitro by antibody produced in syphilis infection. Journal of Experimental Medicine 89: 369-393 (1949).

O'Neill, P.: A new look at the serology of treponemal disease. British Journal of Venereal Disease 52: 296-299 (1976).

Pusch, A.L.: Serodiagnostic tests for syphilis and other diseases; in Davidsohn and Henry (Eds) Clinical Diagnosis by Laboratory Methods, p.1216-1238 (Saunders, Philadelphia 1974).

Further Reading

Sparling, P.F.: Diagnosis and treatment of syphilis. New England Journal of Medicine 284: 642-653 (1971).

Chapter X

Immunoglobulins

1. Immunoglobulin Structure

Immunoglobulins are glycoprotein molecules which have antibody properties. They form the bulk of the gamma globulin fraction of plasma, comprise about 20% of the total plasma proteins, and can also be detected in beta and alpha-2 fractions.

The basic structure of the immunoglobulin molecule consists of two heavy (H) and two light (L) polypeptide chains (fig. 1). The H chains (446 aminoacids) are joined to each other by disulphide bonds. The L chains (214 aminoacids) are united alongside the H chains by sulphydryl bonds. The molecule can bend and revolve at a hinge region.

The portions of the H chains below the hinge form the Fc region and regulate the function of the molecule. The opposite end of the molecule comprises two Fab or antibody combining sites shared by the H and L chains.

The H chains dictate the class and function of the molecule.

2. Functions of Different Immunoglobulins

Immunoglobulins can be divided into classes and sub-classes according to the antigenic properties of the constant regions of the H chains.

There have been 5 classes of immunoglobulins described in humans: immunoglobulin G (IgG), immunoglobulin A (IgA), immunoglobulin M (IgM), immunoglobulin D (IgD) and immunoglobulin E (IgE). Some have been further divided into sub-classes.

There are two distinct antigenic types of L chain termed kappa (k) and lambda (λ) but each immunoglobulin molecule has L chains of only one class.

2.1 Immunoglobulin G (IgG)

This accounts for 73% of the immunoglobulin in normal serum. It is divided into 4 distinctive sub-classes each of which is under separate genetic control. These are termed IgG_1 to IgG_4 and their approximate proportions are: IgG_1 60 to 70%, IgG_2 14 to 20%, IgG_3 4 to 8% and IgG_4 2 to 6%.

Although the individual functions of each sub-class are not fully understood it is known that IgG_1 and IgG_3 fix complement. As IgG_1 is the predominant sub-class it seems likely that the properties ascribed to IgG are probably determined, to a large extent, by this fraction. IgG antibodies seem to arise mainly in response to soluble antigens such as bacterial toxins and they usually appear following an initial response by IgM antibodies. IgG antibodies appear to control the neutralisation of the soluble products which diffuse away from invading organisms. During pregnancy the molecule can pass via the placenta to the fetus.

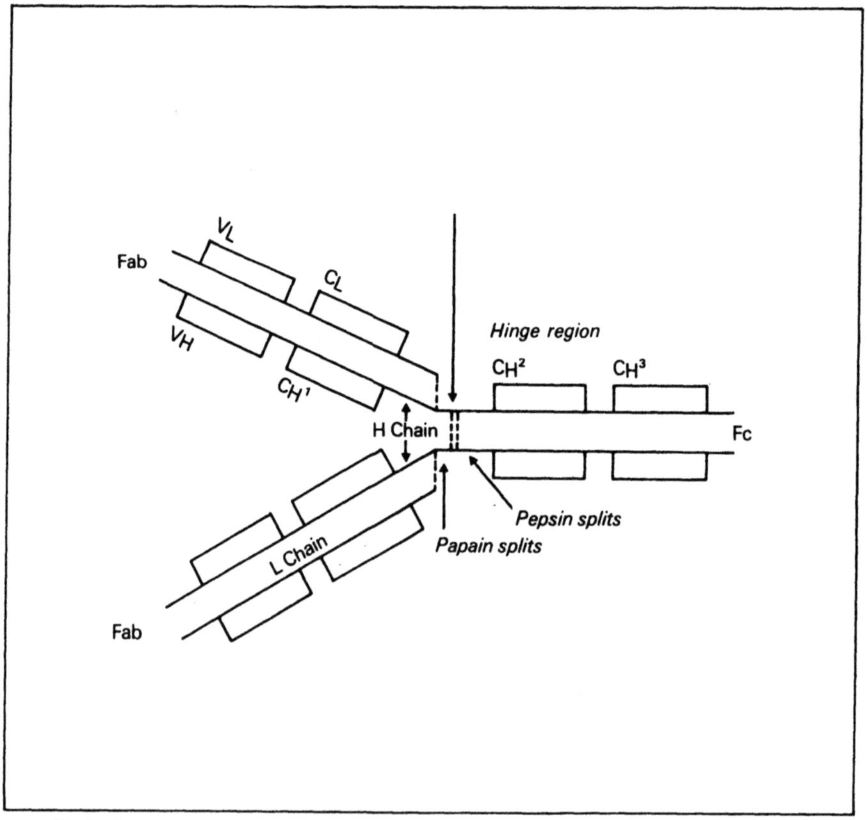

Fig. 1. Structure of the immunoglobulin molecule.

2.2 Immunoglobulin M (IgM)

IgM has a low serum level (approximately 7% of normal serum immunoglobulin) but it appears to have a powerful ability to destroy the surfaces of foreign antigens, especially particulate antigens, in the blood stream. Because of its large size (MW 1,000,000) IgM is restricted to the circulatory system and any IgM found elsewhere, e.g. tissue, joints, CSF, must be manufactured *in situ*.

Although it appears that the principal function of IgM is to protect the circulation, it is considered to have a subsidiary role in the humoral defence of the gut.

2.3 Immunoglobulin A (IgA) and Secretory Immunoglobulin A

IgA constitutes approximately 15% of total serum immunoglobulin but, because it has a fast turnover, its daily synthesis almost equals that of IgG. The major synthesising sites of IgA are the laminae propriae under the mucous membrane of the gut and respiratory tract. IgA has been shown to be the major immunoglobulin in human saliva.

The IgA found in secretions has an additional carbohydrate fraction which is called the secretory piece. This secretory piece protects IgA against the action of digestive enzymes. Secretory IgA can be found in the gut right through to the faeces. It seems to be a vital defence mechanism in the gut where it acts on enteroviruses such as poliomyelitis. Secretory IgA has the ability to fix complement whereas serum IgA does not.

The function of non-secretory IgA is not fully understood but it has been postulated that it may be the major defence mechanism against certain viruses.

2.4 Immunoglobulin E (IgE)

IgE comprises only 0.004% of total serum immunoglobulin but has been shown to be of major importance in allergic diseases. IgE antibodies bind to the membrane of mast cells and basophils in capillaries, skin and tissues of the nasopharynx and bronchi. After an allergen has become bound to the antibodies, the complex triggers the release from mast cells of vasoactive amines, e.g. histamine. This produces a local immediate hypersensitivity reaction such as seen in rhinitis or a generalised reaction as in anaphylaxis.

In *summary,* IgG protects the body fluids, IgA protects the body surfaces and IgM provides initial protection especially to the intravascular system. IgE mediates reaginic hypersensitivity. The function of IgD is unknown but it may play a role in regulating tolerance.

3. Techniques for Measuring Immunoglobulin Levels

A number of different methods of measuring immunoglobulin concentration are available. All the assays described below depend on the same basic principle, that antigen mixed with antibody at equivalent concentrations will precipitate from solution. By standardising the test system with fixed amounts of antibody it is possible to measure the concentration of antigen (in this case immunoglobulin) in the serum, or other solution.

3.1 Immunodiffusion by Plates

This is known as single radial diffusion. Radial diffusion is based on the principle that a quantitative relationship exists between the amount of antigen placed in a well cut in an agar-antibody plate and the resulting ring of precipitation.

The most important use of this technique is in measuring serum immunoglobulin levels. To do this, a monospecific antiserum directed only at Fc or H chain determinants of the immunoglobulin molecule is added to the agar.

This technique is mainly used to detect the higher concentration immunoglobulins, IgG, IgA and IgM; however, 'low-level' plates are made which have increased sensitivity and these can be used to detect IgD, IgE and immunoglobulin levels in immunodeficient patients.

3.2 Electroimmunodiffusion (Rocket Electrophoresis or Laurell Technique)

Antiserum to the antigen that is to be measured is incorporated in an agarose-supporting medium on a glass slide. The specimen to be tested is placed in a small well and electrophoresis moves proteins, including the antigen, into the antibody containing agarose. The resulting patterns of immunoprecipitation resemble rockets, hence the term rocket electrophoresis. The total distance of antigen movement for a given antiserum concentration is proportional to the antigen concentration.

3.3 Nephelometry

Anti-immunoglobulin sera are added to a diluted solution of serum. The antisera and immunoglobulin interact forming complexes which increase the turbidity of the solution. Changes in turbidity are then read in a fluorimeter or nephelometer and compared with a standard. The technique is fast and simple but demands high quality antisera.

Table I. Normal serum immunoglobulin values

Age	IgG		IgA		IgM	
	mg/100ml	IU/ml	mg/100ml	IU/ml	mg/100ml	IU/ml
Newborn	700-1200	80-140	0-12	0-7	5-20	6-25
1-3 months	300-700	35-80	10-40	6-24	15-60	17-70
4-6 months	300-800	35-80	15-50	9-30	20-70	23-80
7-12 months	400-900	45-100	20-60	12-35	25-120	28-140
13-24 months	500-1000	60-115	25-75	15-45	30-130	35-150
25-36 months	600-1200	70-140	35-100	20-60	35-140	40-160
3-5 years	650-1300	75-150	50-130	30-78	40-150	45-170
6-8 years	650-1300	75-150	60-170	35-100	40-150	45-170
9-11 years	700-1400	80-160	70-200	40-120	50-180	60-200
12-16 years	750-1500	85-170	100-230	60-140	50-180	60-200
Adult	800-1600	90-185	150-300	90-180	70-200	80-230

3.4 Electrophoresis

In 1937 Tiselius, using free or moving boundary zone electrophoresis perfected the technique of separating proteins in an electric field. Now zone electrophoresis, which utilises a stabilising medium, such as paper or cellulose acetate, has superseded the original method (Stites, 1978).

3.5 Zone Electrophoresis

Proteins can be separated in zone electrophoresis on the basis of their surface charge. It is presumed that the supporting medium is inert and does not interfere with the flow of molecules in the electrical field.

Serum or other fluid to be tested is placed at the origin and separated by electrophoresis for about 90 minutes using alkaline buffer solutions. Next, the strips are stained and scanned. Scanning changes the band pattern into peaks and in normal human serum 5 bands are seen, gammaglobulin being one.

4. Serum Concentrations of Immunoglobulins

Maternal IgG is transmitted to the fetus across the placenta and then breaks down in the child after birth. Synthesis of immunoglobulin begins in the third trimester and shortly after birth (fig. 2) but the synthetic rates differ for the various immunoglobulin classes. Table I shows the normal serum levels of IgM, IgG and IgA at different ages.

5. Immunoglobulin Levels in Disease

In disease immunoglobulin levels may be either increased or decreased.

5.1 Immunoglobulin Deficiencies

These may arise from:
1) Defective synthesis
2) Increased loss from the body
3) Increased catabolism.

Defective synthesis

Immunoglobulin levels in the serum depend upon rates of synthesis, rates of catabolism, and the extent of immunoglobulin loss from the body. Depressed im-

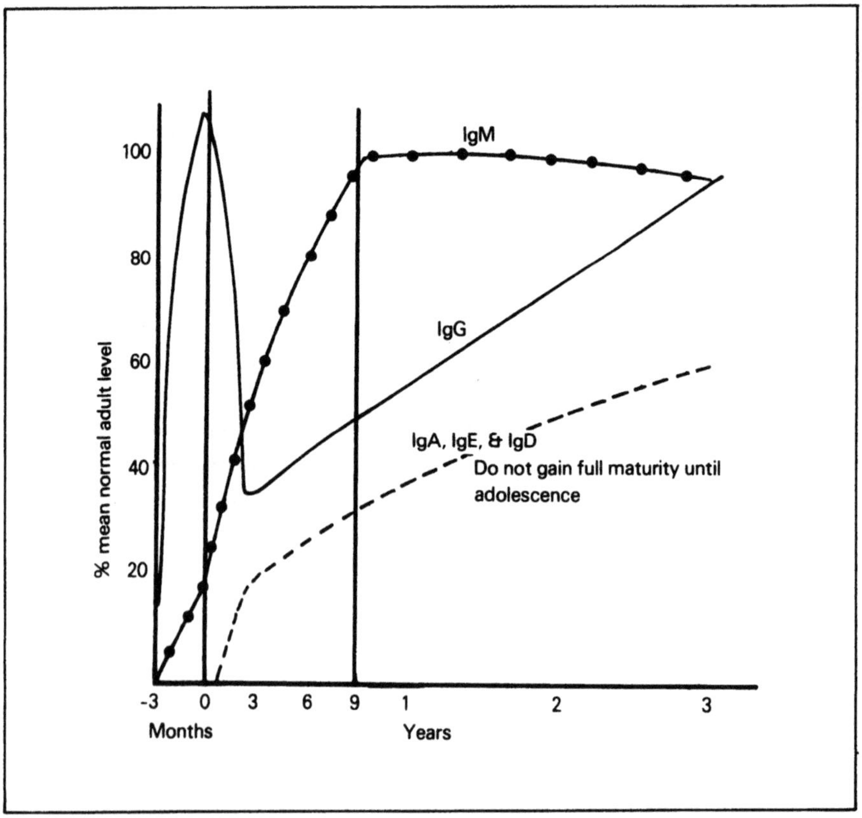

Fig. 2. Changing antibody levels with age. From Hobbs (1971) with permission of the author.

Table II. The causes of pathological loss of immunoglobulins

Gastrointestinal tract (protein-losing gastroenteropathy)
Ulcerative colitis
GI tract carcinoma
Coeliac disease
Whipple's disease
Lymphoma
Intestinal lymphangiectasia
Constrictive pericarditis
Tricuspid incompetence
Kidney (nephrotic syndrome)
Glomerulonephritis (minimal change, membranous, proliferative)
Renal vein thrombosis
Diabetes
Amyloidosis
Systemic lupus erythematosus
Lymphomas
Skin
Acute burns
Atopic dermatitis
Peritoneum
Recurrent removal of ascitic fluid

munoglobulin levels may arise because of primary and secondary defects in synthesis which are discussed in chapter XXI.

Increased Immunoglobulin Loss

Table II summarises conditions where immunoglobulin molecules are lost from the body. The most common of these causes of declining serum immunoglobulin levels are the nephrotic syndrome and burns. IgG is preferentially depleted in the nephrotic syndrome and the decline is accelerated by increased catabolism of immunoglobulins. A selective loss of L chains can occur in patients with renal disease from SLE.

Following major burns all immunoglobulin classes decline rapidly over 2 to 3 days. Levels of IgM recover within 7 to 10 days and IgA and IgG over the following week. IgG may fall below 2.0g/litre, the lowest levels occurring in patients with lethal burns. Decreased immunoglobulin synthesis, and increased catabolism, contribute to the lowered immunoglobulin levels but the major loss is from exudation from the burns.

With protein-losing gastroenteropathy the protein loss is non-selective and all immunoglobulin classes decline. In addition lymphocytes are lost from the gut surface and lymphopenia often results.

Increased Immunoglobulin Catabolism

A number of rare conditions are associated with decreased immunoglobulin levels from increased catabolism. These include Wiskott-Aldrich syndrome, myotonic dystrophy and ataxia telangiectasia. In thyrotoxicosis and Cushing's disease immunoglobulin may be depressed as part of a generalised increase in protein catabolism.

5.2 Increased Immunoglobulin Levels

Polyclonal Gammopathy

An increased gammaglobulin band in an electrophorectic analysis of a patient's serum is a common finding. This indicates a generalised increase in the patient's immunoglobulins, usually involving all classes, and can arise with any of a number of different disorders including chronic infections and autoimmune diseases such as SLE, rheumatoid arthritis and chronic liver disease. The information below is provided as a guide to situations where increased gammaglobulins are found, and offers some diagnostic aids by showing where one or more immunoglobulin classes are selectively raised.

In many situations all immunoglobulin classes are raised but one class exhibits a greater change than the others. This will be described below as dominant elevation of the class most affected.

Diseases of the liver: As a general rule:

1) Dominant elevation of IgM occurs with primary biliary cirrhosis and is also found soon after the onset of acute hepatitis.
2) Dominant elevation of IgG occurs with chronic aggressive hepatitis and a less striking elevation of IgG can be seen after the initial IgM response in acute hepatitis.
3) Dominant elevation of IgA occurs with the Laennec type of cirrhosis.
4) With other diseases affecting the liver a nonspecific pattern can be seen. Diseases showing this are secondary biliary cirrhosis, sarcoidosis, tuberculosis, and late mixed cirrhosis.

Cardiovascular disease: 95% of patients with active rheumatic fever show an elevation of IgA and IgG, and in patients with untreated bacterial endocarditis IgG, IgA and IgM levels rise in about equal amounts.

Respiratory diseases: A number of respiratory diseases, particularly bronchial asthma, are associated with a dominant IgE elevation so this has no specific diagnostic value. In infants, *Pneumocystis pneumonia* can elevate IgM.

Table III. Classification of paraproteinaemias. From Wells and Ries (1978) with permission of the authors

Malignant monoclonal gammopathy	Monocytic leukaemia
Multiple myeloma	Rheumatoid disorders
Waldenstrom's macroglobulinaemia	Chronic inflammatory states
Solitary plasmacytoma	Cold agglutinin syndrome
Amyloidosis	Papular mucinosis
Heavy chain diseases	Immunodeficiency
Malignant lymphoma	
Chronic lymphocytic leukaemia	*Benign monoclonal gammopathy*
	Transient
Secondary monoclonal gammopathy	Persistent
Cancer (non-lymphoreticular)	

Gut diseases: Although the presence of raised IgA when associated with malabsorption states has little diagnostic value, the persistence of a high IgA level seems to indicate a continuing disease activity.

Renal disease: The interpretation of serum immunoglobulin levels in renal disease is complicated on two counts: immunoglobulins are lost in the urine with proteinuria and a toxic inhibition of synthesis can occur affecting primarily IgM, then IgA and lastly IgG.

Skin diseases: Most skin diseases evoke some IgA elevation and usually the more extensive the lesions the higher the IgA level. It can be presumed from this that IgA plays a protective role in defence of the skin. In dermatomyositis there is marked IgA elevation. Psoriasis and dermatitis herpetiformis patients often show depressed IgM levels. Atopic dermatitis (eczema) is associated with high IgM levels.

6. Paraproteinaemias

A paraprotein (or M protein) is a homogeneous protein appearing in an electrophoretic strip of a patient's serum as a dense narrow band. It represents an immunoglobulin produced by a single clone of plasma cells. Although associated with a number of different conditions the importance of detecting a paraprotein lies in the fact that in many cases it results from a malignant expansion of plasma cells — multiple myeloma or macroglobulinaemia. Approximately 0.2 % of the population will have a paraprotein. The prevalence increases with age and paraproteins are found in up to 0.6 % of people over the age of 60 (Carter, 1977). Some surveys have found paraproteins in up to 8 % of patients older than 70 (Wells and Ries, 1978). In most cases when paraproteins are detected by chance the patient has a benign condition. However, rising concentrations of the paraprotein indicate a probable malignant origin. A classification of clinical conditions associated with paraproteins is given in table III.

50% of paraproteins are IgG and 25% IgA; IgD and IgM paraproteins are uncommon while IgE paraproteins are very rare. Some patients have very high levels of free kappa or lambda light chains. When free light chains appear in the urine they constitute Bence-Jones protein.

Diagnostic markers suggesting a malignant origin of the paraprotein include the patient's history, the physical findings of tumour (including bone marrow), x-ray changes of myeloma, rising levels of the paraprotein with time and low levels of the normal immunoglobulins. The last mentioned finding is characteristic of almost all patients with myeloma and can be identified by measuring the individual immunoglobulin levels whenever a paraprotein is detected.

6.1 Complications from Paraproteins

Hyperviscosity Syndrome

When paraprotein concentrations reach very high levels, particularly with IgM, symptoms can appear from the increased viscosity of the patient's blood. Cardiac failure, breathlessness and haemorrhages can occur.

Cryoglobulinaemia

Cryoglobulins are serum proteins which precipitate at low temperatures. Under some circumstances they may precipitate intravascularly producing a variety of symptoms ranging from Raynaud's phenomenon to purpura, nephritis and arthritis. Once a cryoglobulin has been identified there are strong clinical indications to characterise it as the different forms are associated with different clinical conditions.

Type I cryoglobulins: These represent high concentrations of monoclonal globulins which will cryoprecipitate if their concentration is high enough. Most are of the IgM class rather than IgG or IgA and they are almost always a product of macroglobulinaemia or myeloma. Raynaud's phenomenon and vascular occlusion are the commonest symptoms.

Type II cryoglobulins: Some monoclonal paraproteins have rheumatoid factor activity and these can combine with IgM acquiring the capacity to cryoprecipitate. This form of cryoglobulin is most commonly of the IgM class and is found associated with macroglobulinanaemia and various lymphomas. Purpura and vasculitis are the predominant clinical features.

Type III cryoglobulins: Polyclonal cryoglobulins normally of the IgM and IgG classes can occur. Together with the Type II form they constitute 'mixed', in contrast to monoclonal, cryoglobulins. They occur in patients with autoimmune diseases (in particular those with a high prevalence of rheumatoid factor) and will appear transiently in patients with some infections. About one-third of patients with cryoglobulins have no underlying disease although the presence of the cryoglobulin may precede clinical signs of malignancy by up to 10 years.

When sufficient cryoglobulin is present it can be precipitated *in vitro* and analysed immunochemically to establish its monoclonal or mixed character. This provides clear clinical guidelines to the possible associated diseases.

6.2 Diseases Associated with Paraproteinaemia

Multiple Myeloma

Almost 80% of patients with myeloma have paraproteins in their serum but occasional patients have malignant plasma cells which are not secreting immunoglobulins and thus lack a serum paraprotein. The remaining patients have free L chains in their urine detectable immunochemically and which represent Bence-Jones protein. Bence-Jones protein is also present in many of the patients with serum paraproteins.

Following their diagnosis patients can be monitored by following the concentration of their paraprotein. Almost invariably normal immunoglobulins are decreased in these patients. There are slight differences in prognosis depending on the class of the paraproteins. Patients with IgG myeloma have the best prognosis, then those with IgA myeloma, while the poorest survival rate is found with Bence-Jones myeloma.

Macroglobulinaemia

Hyperviscosity is the major complication for those patients with high concentrations of IgM paraproteins.

Other Lymphomas

Occasionally lymphomas or chronic lymphytic leukaemia are associated with paraprotein, presumably because their malignant lymphocytes are secreting immunoglobulin.

6.3 Benign Paraproteins

In some patients levels of the paraprotein will remain constant for many years and this is representative of benign non-progressive paraproteinaemia. In these cases, in contrast to the situation in myeloma, the M protein concentration is usually less than 2.0g/litre, the patient is usually elderly and other immunoglobulin levels are not reduced.

In a few patients a paraprotein will appear transiently for a few weeks or months, and then disappear, and this is often related to a viral infection.

References

Carter, P.: Monoclonal proteins; in Holborow and Reeves (Eds) Immunology in Medicine p.957-997 (Academic Press, London 1977).

Hobbs, J.R.: Immunoglobulins in clinical chemistry. Advances in Clinical Chemistry 14: 219-317 (1971).

Laurell, C.B.: Antigen-antibody crossed electrophoresis. Analytical Biochemistry 10: 358-361 (1965).

Stites, D.P.: Clinical laboratory methods for detection of antigens and antibodies; in Fudenberg, Stites, Caldwell and Wells (Eds) Basic and Clinical Immunology, p.337-374 (Lange Medical Publications, California 1978).

Wells, J.V. and Ries, C.A.: Haematologic diseases; in Fudenberg, Stites, Caldwell and Wells (Eds) Basic and Clinical Immunology, p.452-500 (Lange Medical Publications, California 1978)

Further Reading

McKelvey, E.M. and Fahey, J.L.: Immunoglobulin changes in disease: quantitation on the basis of heavy polypeptide chains, IgG (γG), IgA (γA) and IgM (γM) and of light peptide chains, type K (I) and type L (II). Journal of Clinical Investigation 44: 1778-1787 (1965).

Chapter XI

Complement

Complement is a collective term for a complex series of proteins and enzymes which play an important role in antibody-directed body defences. Analysis of selected complement components provides clinical information of value in the diagnosis of some conditions and acts as a laboratory index of disease activity and recovery.

There are a number of components in the human complement system numbered from 1 to 9, e.g. C3, C4. C1 is formed of 3 separate sub-units C1q, C1r, C1s. The individual components interact together in a complex sequence (fig. 1) similar to the cascade system of blood coagulation. Initiation of this cascade (activation or fixation of complement) occurs with the union of antibody with antigen to form an immune complex. When such a complex is added to serum *in vitro* or *in vivo,* the complement components react with the complex in a consistent sequence. The rate of reaction is modulated both by the instability of certain complement enzymes and by the presence in serum of control proteins that act as inhibitors or inactivators.

As complement is activated in this way the various components are consumed and must be replaced by fresh synthesis. Serum levels of complement fall:

1) If consumption outstrips synthesis, as with very active antibody-antigen interaction
2) When synthesis falls, as in advanced liver disease
3) When C3 nephritic factor develops which continually breaks down C3.

On occasions, as with some other serum proteins, levels of some complement components may rise during acute inflammation, particularly with acute arthritis. Only antibodies of IgM, IgG_1 and IgG_3 classes fix complement.

An alternate pathway for activation of complement exists and this is initiated by aggregates of some immunoglobulins, by bacterial endotoxins and by some polysaccharides such as inulin and zymosan.

1. Biological Role of Complement

Antibodies identify foreign antigens which are then disposed of by various mechanisms including phagocytosis and the complement system. For example antibody-coated bacteria may happily survive until exposed to complement, when they are lysed. There are a number of different activities mediated by complement.

1.1 Immune Lysis

The activity of complement which has been most intensely investigated is its function in immune lysis. The role of complement in this bactericidal reaction was one of the first recognised functions of complement. A number of Gram-negative bacteria, including Salmonella, Escherichia, Shigella, Brucella, Proteus, Haemophilus

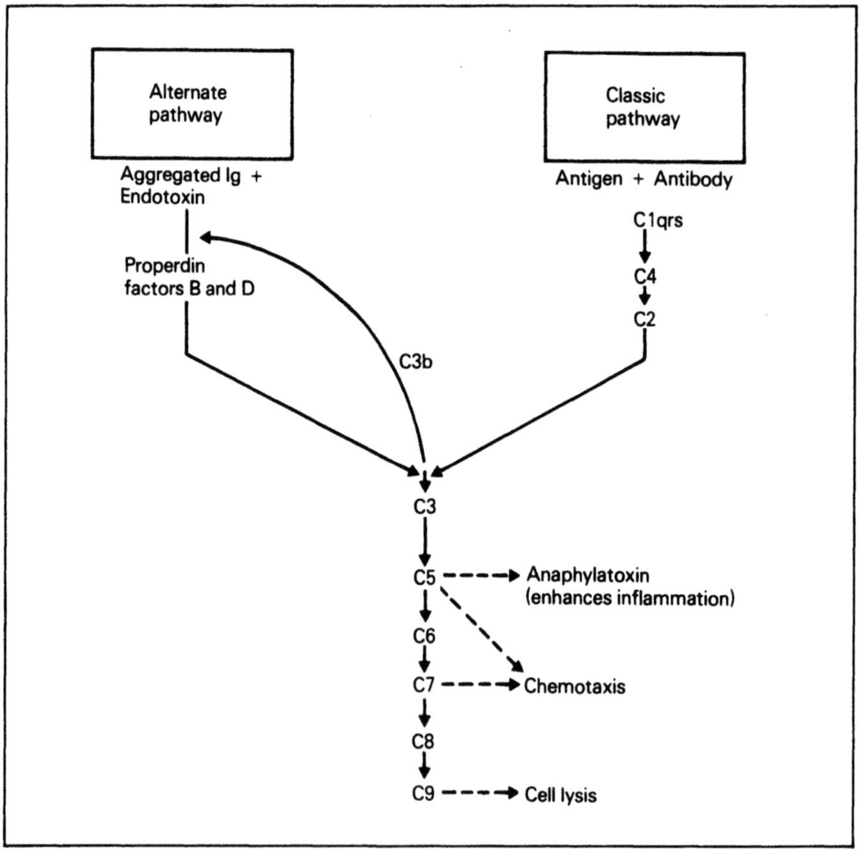

Fig. 1. Reactions which occur during complement activation.

and Vibrio are killed by the action of antibody and complement. Gram-positive organisms are usually resistant to the cytotoxic action of complement although they may be destroyed by complement-dependent phagocytosis. Complement in conjunction with antibody appears to act upon certain protozoa and spirochaetes, and also neutralises viruses in various ways.

1.2 Complement as a Permeability Increasing Factor

The first component of complement may be activated by an immune complex to the enzymatic state of C1 esterase. It has been suggested that this enzyme is capable of increasing vascular permeability (Thompson, 1977).

1.3 Phagocytosis

Phagocytosis is enhanced following immune adherence of antigens to phagocytes and is dependent upon the third component of complement. Erythrophagocytosis is also a complement-dependent reaction.

1.4 Inflammation

Various active fractions of complement (anaphylatoxins) enhance local inflammation.

1.5 Chemotaxis

It has been shown recently that complement in combination with an immune complex results in the liberation of a powerful polymorphonuclear leukocyte chemotactic factor (Ruddy et al., 1972).

1.6 Arthus Reaction

Bound complement has been found in Arthus lesions and it appears that this acute inflammatory condition is mediated by components of complement, possibly C1, C4, C2 and C3.

2. Complement Assays

Because of the complexity of the complement system and the apparently different biological role of each component of the complement system, a number of different assays are necessary. The principles of these tests are discussed.

2.1 Haemolytic Complement CH_{50}

Antibody-sensitised red cells are mixed with the patient's serum *in vitro*. The red cells lyse with complement from the added serum. Using various dilutions of serum, a quantitative measure of the complement levels is obtained and is expressed as CH_{50} units/ml (1 unit = amount of complement to lyse 5×10^7 antibody-sensitised sheep red cells under standard conditions). Depression of individual complement components will usually be reflected in low CH_{50} units (normal values 80 to 140u/ml). Individual laboratories may have varied ways of expressing results and different normal values.

2.2 Individual Complement Components

Although assays are available for all complement components, those most commonly measured are C1q, C3 and C4. Immunodiffusion is the standard method and results are expressed in mg/100ml or g/litre. Normal values are:

C1q 17 to 20mg/100ml 0.17 to 0.2g/litre
C3 80 to 140mg/100ml 0.8 to 1.4g/litre
C4 20 to 50mg/100ml 0.2 to 0.5g/litre.

Individual laboratories may have a slightly different normal range.

2.3 Anticomplementary Activity

This is the capacity of serum to inhibit complement's function *in vitro* and usually indicates the presence of circulating antigen-antibody complexes. It therefore acts as a direct indication of disease activity in immune complex diseases such as SLE. The levels are described by the laboratory as being increased or within their normal limits.

2.4 C3 Breakdown Products

Some specialist laboratories can estimate C3 breakdown products which are the forms of C3 produced following activation of the complement sequence. These forms (C3c and C3d) are usually detected by crossed immunoelectrophoresis and are a direct indication of *in vivo* complement activation. Results are expressed as C3 breakdown products — within normal limits or increased. Eventually it should be possible to measure C3c and C3d directly and express results as g/litre.

2.5 C1 Esterase Inhibitor

This regulator component is estimated by standard immunodiffusion or by a more complicated functional assay. Normal levels are 0.03 to 0.5g/litre (immunodiffusion).

3. Evaluation of Complement Tests

A number of alterations in the complement system occur clinically. These include altered rate of synthesis or catabolism, absence of one or more components, and a generalised rise or fall of serum levels of some components. Depressed complement levels almost always indicate disease. The only exception occurs with total complement measured by the haemolytic CH_{50} assay, as titres may fall in serum left on the bench for some hours or days. In this circumstance C3 and C4 levels will not fall. The clinical course of patients with depressed complement can usually be monitored critically by following complement levels.

Tables I and II are a guide to conditions where complement levels are altered. Normal complement levels do not exclude any diagnosis as increased synthesis can replace complement which is consumed by antigen-antibody reactions. It has been shown, where methods for detection of complement breakdown products (particularly C3c and C3d) are available, that a rise in these products indicates increased *in vivo* complement consumption, even when complement levels are normal (McKay, personal communication).

The complexity of the complement system demands the application of a number of tests to assist interpretation.

4. Complement Changes in Human Disease

4.1 Inborn Errors

4.1.1 Deficiencies of Complement Components

These rare conditions are usually familial. Their interest lies in the fact that a deficiency of any complement component is usually (but not always) associated with clear clinical manifestations, principally recurrent infections or autoimmune disease.

Table II lists the recognised complement deficiencies. The commonest are C2 and various forms of C3 deficiency. C2 deficiency is inherited as an autosomal recessive trait and while some patients are entirely healthy others develop SLE. Both heterozygous and homozygous forms can be detected.

4.1.2 Hereditary Angioneurotic Oedema

C1 esterase inhibitor is an important regulator of the complement system and a deficiency is inherited as an autosomal dominant trait (Hadjyannaki and Lachman,

Table I. Classification of complement changes in human diseases

Inborn errors
Deficiencies of complement components
Hereditary angioneurotic oedema
Acquired abnormalities
Elevation of complement
Depression of complement
in vivo activation
decreased synthesis
C3 nephritic factor

Table II. Hereditary deficiencies of complement components. Adapted with permission of the authors from Thaler et al. (1977)

Complement component deficient	Clinical features
C1q	Hypogammaglobulinaemia and severe combined immune deficiency
C1r	Recurrent infections, glomerulonephritis, lupus-like syndrome
C1s	Seen in 1 patient with SLE
C2	Increased incidence SLE. Some patients healthy
C3	Increased infections
C4	Lupus-like syndrome
C5	Lupus-like syndrome, recurrent infections
C6	No disease
C7	1 patient with scleroderma
C8	1 patient with disseminated *N. gonorrhoea* infection
C1 esterase inhibitor	Hereditary angioneurotic oedema

1971). This is expressed clinically as recurrent episodes of acute circumscribed non-inflammatory oedema of the skin, gastrointestinal tract and the mucosa of the upper respiratory tract. The oedema is not itchy and lasts 2 to 4 days. The patients are at great risk when oedema involves the upper airways as respiratory obstruction can ensue. In about 15% of patients C1 esterase inhibitor levels, determined by immunodiffusion, are normal but complexed to other proteins and can be shown to be abnormal in functional assays or by crossed immunoelectrophoresis. During attacks, C4 and C2 levels fall while C1 and C3 are normal. Between attacks C4 is usually depressed. Accurate diagnosis of this condition is important as medical management is difficult because the patients do not respond to adrenaline, antihistamines or steroids.

4.2 Acquired Abnormalities

4.2.1 Elevated Complement Levels

With acute inflammatory processes the concentrations of various acute-phase proteins increase in the serum. Some complement components are similarly elevated. Increased C4 and C3 have been recorded in acute phases of rheumatic fever, periarteritis nodosa, dermatomyositis, myocardial infarction, typhoid fever, gout, Reiter's syndrome and various forms of polyarthritis. The reaction results from increased complement synthesis.

4.2.2 Depressed Complement Levels

Serum levels of various complement components may be depressed by one or more of the following mechanisms:

1) Where an antigen-antibody reaction is sufficiently extensive serum complement levels fall until synthesis matches consumption. Classically this is all or part of the explanation for the low complement levels in SLE.

2) Most complement components are synthesised in the liver and generalised liver disease may be associated with low complement levels from decreased synthesis.

3) Various complement components may be inactivated or consumed by the action of various non-complement factors. A serum factor (C3 nephritic factor) appears in some forms of renal disease e.g. mesangio capillary glomerulonephritis and acute glomerulonephritis. This factor inactivates C3, and serum complement levels fall. In some instances of tissue injury — trauma, severe infections or ischaemia — various proteolytic enzymes may be released which cleave various complement components and thus decrease their serum level.

Depression of serum complement levels, by any of the above mechanisms, indicates pathology. The major value in identifying this phenomenon is firstly to assist in diagnosis and secondly, having shown low complement in a patient, to use this as an index of the patient's progress. Because complement is subject to the effect of antigen-antibody formation and of altered synthesis, changing complement levels in patients provide more clinical information than one isolated determination.

4.3 Conditions Frequently Associated with Depressed Complement Levels

4.3.1 Poststreptococcal Acute Glomerulonephritis

In most cases complement falls to very low levels within the first days of the illness. CH_{50} and C3 are most depressed. C4 may be normal or increased, particularly in the early stages of the inflammatory process.

Table III. Conditions associated with anticomplementary activity in a proportion of patients

Acute post-streptococcal glomerulonephritis
Active phases of SLE
Acute hepatitis B (prodromal stages only)
Immune complex-induced vasculitis during active phases
Brucellosis — during early stages of acute infections
Dermatitis herpetiformis
Primary biliary cirrhosis
Active secondary syphilis
Some acute bacterial and viral infections
Myelomatosis and macroglobulinaemia
Chronic active hepatitis

4.3.2 Acute Phases of Systemic Lupus Erythematosus

In most patients CH_{50}, C3 and C4 will be depressed during active phases. Although complement is a valuable index of disease activity there are circumstances in which *in vivo* complement activation ceases but complement remains low because synthesis is depressed by immunosuppressive therapy or possibly by negative feedback of synthesis. Levels recover as treatment is tailed off.

4.3.3 Chronic Mesangiocapillary Glomerulonephritis

C3 is particularly affected by C3 nephritic factor which is often detectable in the serum.

4.3.4 Acute Viral Hepatitis B

In this disease C4, and to a lesser extent C3, levels may be depressed in the prodromal stages.

4.3.5 Subacute Bacterial Endocarditis

Depressed complement levels occur particularly in patients with associated glomerulonephritis.

4.3.6 Chronic Liver Disease

Both C3 and C4 may be reduced in chronic active hepatitis, primary biliary cirrhosis and advanced cirrhosis.

4.3.7 Rheumatoid Arthritis

Serum complement is reduced in about 10% of the most severely afflicted patients; intra-articular complement is commonly reduced.

4.3.8 Angioneurotic Oedema

C4 levels are reduced in this condition (see 4.1.2).

4.4 Conditions Occasionally Associated with Depressed Complement Levels

1) Autoimmune haemolytic anaemia and cryoglobulinaemia — some patients only
2) Sjogren's syndrome, myeloma, lymphoma, myasthenia gravis — in occasional patients
3) Some acute viral and bacterial infections.

5. Anticomplementary Activity

When *in vivo* antigen-antibody complexes are formed these are usually rapidly cleared by phagocytic cells. Under some circumstances, because of the size of the complexes, their concentration, or their quality, they will remain in the circulation for a time and reveal their presence *in vitro* by anti-complementary activity. If sufficient complex formation has occurred, the patient will exhibit both anti-complementary activity and depressed complement levels. However, anti-complementary activity can occur without alterations in the level of complement components. It must be remembered that not all immune complexes are complement-fixing and so some will not be revealed by this assay. Table III lists some conditions where a proportion of patients will have anti-complementary activity in their serum.

References

Hadjyannaki, K. and Lachman, P.J.: Hereditary angio-oedema: A review with particular reference to pathogenesis and treatment. Clinical Allergy 1: 221-233 (1971).

Ruddy, S.; Gigli, I. and Austen, K.F.: The complement system of man; (4 parts). New England Journal of Medicine 287: 489-495; 545-549; 592-596; 642-646 (1972).

Thaler, M.S.; Klausner, R.D. and Cohen, J.H.: The immunodeficiency diseases; in Medical Immunology, p.237-270 (Lippincott, Philadelphia 1977).

Thompson, R.A.: Complement in perspective; in Holborow and Reeves (Eds) Immunology in Medicine, p.191-229 (Academic Press, London 1977).

Further Reading

Cooper, N.R. and Fogel, B.J.: Complement in normal and disease processes. Journal of Pediatrics 70: 982-996 (1967).

Chapter XII

Autoantibodies

Antibodies that react with various tissue fractions of one's own body are termed autoantibodies. These are being recognised with increasing frequency with the development of immunofluorescent techniques (fig. 1). Although in some cases there are definite associations between a specific antibody and a particular disease (such as antithyroid antibodies in thyroid disease) in other circumstances a disorder restricted to a single organ may be accompanied by an antibody which reacts against tissue from many sites. Often the presence of autoantibodies is not in itself diagnostic and must be considered along with other clinical and laboratory data for each patient.

Some healthy people, particularly older people and especially women, have autoantibodies. There also appears to be a genetic predisposition in some individuals to develop certain diseases associated with autoantibodies.

1. Categories of Antibody

Autoantibodies to different tissues can be considered in three groups.

Group 1: Disease Associated with Organ-specific Antibodies

Antibodies to several organs may be present in these disorders but the antibody against the organ primarily affected is usually in highest titre, e.g. Hashimoto's thyroiditis, pernicious anaemia, idiopathic adrenal insufficiency.

Group 2: Connective Tissue Disorders

In these diseases non-organ-specific antibodies predominate. Antinuclear antibody, rheumatoid factor and collagen antibodies appear in various proportions. The chronic liver diseases such as primary biliary cirrhosis and chronic hepatitis also fall into this category.

Group 3: Antibodies Against Various Formed Elements in the Circulation.

This group includes for example, antibodies to leucocytes and/or platelets and to red cell antigens.

2. Individual Antibodies

2.1 Antinuclear Antibodies (ANA)

These are antibodies directed against various nuclear constituents and they are of particular importance in some autoimmune diseases such as systemic lupus erythematosus (SLE). Increasingly it is recognised that ANA comprise a number of different antibodies with specificity for different nuclear constituents. Antibodies to native double stranded DNA, denatured or single stranded DNA, RNA and nucleoproteins are all detected as ANA by immunofluorescence.

2.1.1 Assay Method

The most satisfactory screening method for ANA is indirect immunofluoroescence (IF). Cryostat cut sections of tissue — rat liver or calf adrenal are commonly used — are placed on a slide. A drop of patient's serum is added and antibody to nuclei, if present, binds to nuclei of the tissue section. The slide is washed and fluores-

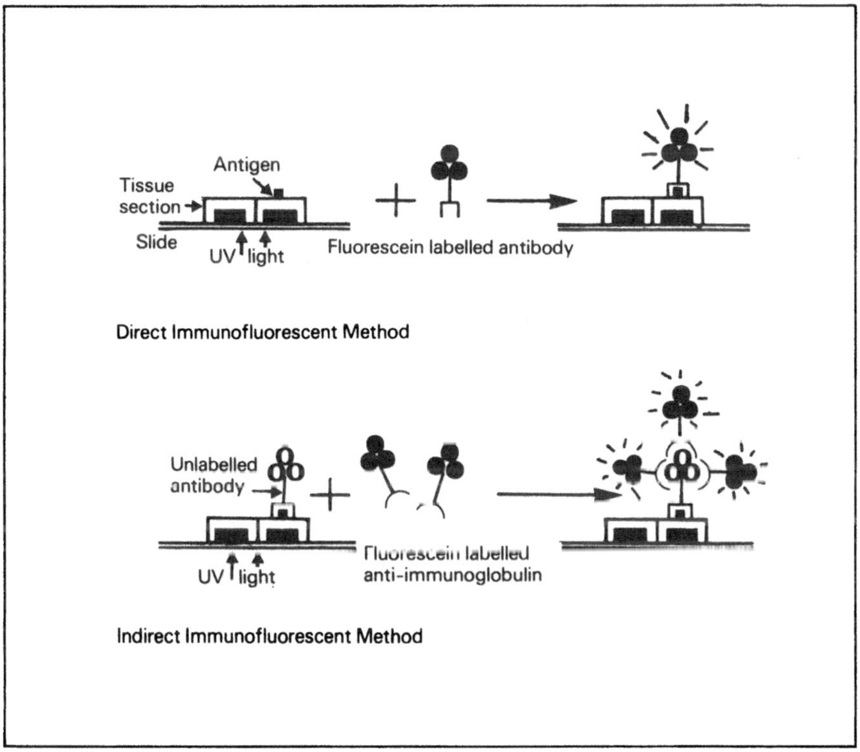

Fig. 1. Immunofluorescent techniques. Adapted from Roitt (1974) with permission of the author.

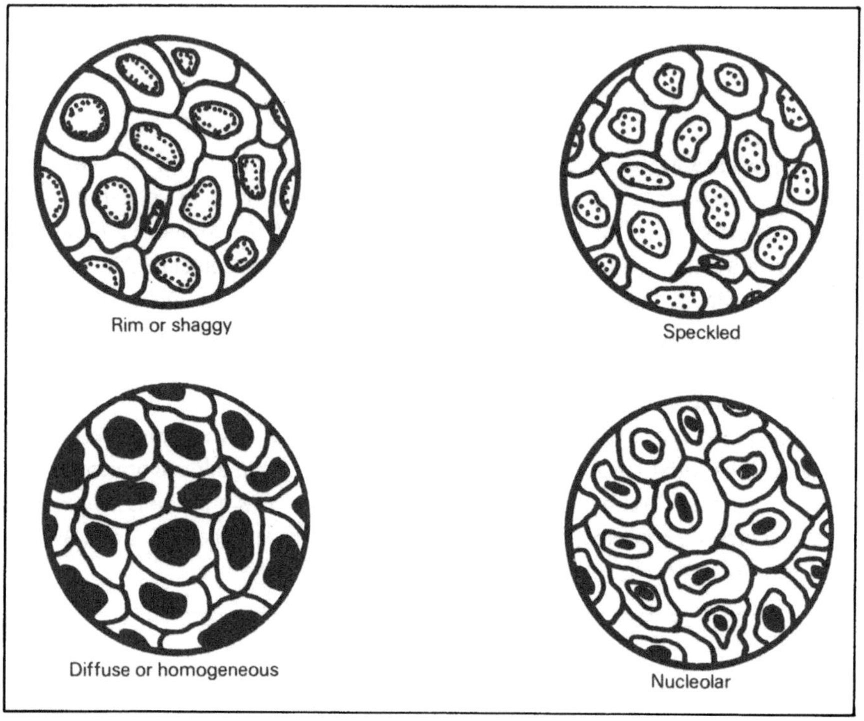

Fig. 2. Different patterns of antinuclear antibody (ANA) immunfluorescent staining.

cein-labelled antibody directed against human immunoglobulin is added. Where ANA is present it is revealed by fluorescence of the tissue nuclei. A number of different patterns of fluorescence are seen — diffuse, speckled, membranous or nucleolar. These are shown in figure 2. It was initially believed that there were clear relationships between individual patterns and particular diseases; however, these relationships have become blurred and greater relevance seems likely to apply to the precise specificity of the antinuclear antibodies, i.e. whether they react with double or single stranded DNA or RNA etcetara (Hughes and Lachman, 1975).

2.1.2 A Guide to the Rough Clinical Correlations of the Different Patterns

The speckled pattern: This is given by antibodies to acidic nucleoproteins. One of these proteins is a nuclear macromolecule, provisionally termed the Sm antigen and another, an acidic ribonucleoprotein which has been termed extractable nuclear antigen (ENA). Speckled pattern staining is seen in about 25 % of patients with SLE, in chronic discoid lupus erythematosus associated with erythema multiforme-like lesions, and in some patients with progressive systemic sclerosis, Sjogren's syndrome and Raynaud's phenomenon.

The nucleolar pattern: This pattern is thought to result from antibody directed against a specific RNA configuration of the nucleolus, or antibody specific for proteins necessary for the maturation of nucleolar RNA. It is seen in patients with scleroderma or SLE.

The homogeneous pattern: The nucleus stains in a diffuse pattern from antibody to deoxyribonucleoprotein. This pattern is present in high titre in most cases of acute SLE.

The peripheral pattern: The antibody responsible for this type of staining (also termed rim, shaggy or membranous) reacts with DNA in the rim of the nucleus and is sometimes found in association with the diffuse pattern. The presence of this antibody in high titre suggests active SLE and usually implies renal involvement. It is found in up to 10% of patients with SLE and is diagnostic of the disease.

2.1.3 Specificity of ANA

A variety of techniques is used to identify the precise antigens to which ANA is directed. Of these the most important are anti-DNA (double stranded) antibody, which is almost pathognomonic for SLE, and antibodies to extractable nuclear antigen (ENA), which is largely ribonucleoprotein, and is present in very high titres in mixed connective tissue disease (MCTD) [Hughes and Lachman, 1975].

2.1.4 Detection of DNA and ENA Antibodies

Antibodies to double stranded (native) and single stranded (denatured) DNA can now be readily detected. Although a large number of techniques are available those in most common use are the Farr test, the Crithidia assay and haemagglutination.

The Farr test: This test employs radio-labelled DNA which, when mixed with serum containing DNA antibody, forms a complex of antibody with labelled DNA antigen. Antibody in the serum is then precipitated with the addition of ammonium sulphate. Where anti-DNA antibody is present the radio-labelled DNA will be precipitated as well for it is bound to the antibody. The result is expressed as percent labelled DNA precipitated. Normal values are usually less than 20% precipitated and in people with very active SLE up to 98% of the DNA will be precipitated in this test (Hughes and Lachman, 1975). It is technically very difficult and from time to time a laboratory's normal values will change.

Crithidia assay: This assay uses a micro-organism *(Crithidia)* which contains a concentration of DNA in an organelle termed a kinetoplast. Anti-DNA antibodies are detected by indirect immunofluorescence when slides of the *Crithidia* are coated with the patient's serum from which anti-DNA antibodies will bind to the kinetoplasts. The washed slides are then labelled with fluorescent labelled anti-human immunoglobulin and a positive result is seen where the kinetoplast of the organism is fluorescing. Positive responses are found more frequently with the Crithidia assay than with the Farr assay because the former is more sensitive.

Metaphase assay: A recent development has been the use of human chromosome preparations as substrate for an immunofluoresence assay for DNA antibodies. Results are similar to those obtained with Crithidia.

Haemagglutination: If very carefully purified, both double and single stranded DNA can be tagged to the surface of red cells so that in the presence of DNA antibody the reaction can be visualised by agglutination of the red cells. At present the major technical difficulty of this technique is to obtain double stranded DNA almost completely free of single stranded DNA. Results are expressed as a titre of anti-DNA antibody.

It may take a few years before the relative value of each of these assays in the diagnosis and management of SLE is fully established. Consequently it is probably worthwhile running all 5 of these assays for each investigation.

During an active phase of their disease most patients with SLE will develop double stranded anti-DNA antibodies. These occur in very few other conditions and provide a good guide to disease activity. Some patients with chronic active hepatitis also have anti-double-stranded DNA antibodies but their occurrence outside these two conditions is very rare.

Antibody to Extractable Nuclear Antigens (ENA)

Antibody to ENA is detected by a haemagglutination method. Of greater clinical importance is antiribonucleoprotein antibody which can also be assayed by indirect IF and confirmed using RNAse-treated tissue sections.

Detection of antibody to ENA with a non-defined specificity allows recognition of the syndrome termed mixed connective tissue disease (MCTD) which is characterised by an excellent response to corticosteroid therapy and a favourable prognosis. 100% of patients with MCTD show high titre speckled fluorescent antinuclear antibody (Sharp et al., 1972). There is no detectable smooth muscle antibody, and antibody to native DNA occurs in low titre in about 30% of patients. Serum complement levels are normal or elevated. Patients with MCTD have clinical features which overlap with SLE, scleroderma and dermatomyositis. They have arthritis and arthralgia, Raynaud's phenomenon, myositis, lymphadenopathy, serositis, splenomegaly, anaemia, leukopenia and hypergammaglobulinaemia. Renal disease is present in 5 to 10% of these patients.

It is obvious that by clinical criteria alone a diagnosis of SLE, scleroderma or myositis in such a patient is difficult to make. The distinguishing feature is the presence in MCTD of high titres of ANA to ribonucleoprotein. Recognition of these cases of scleroderma and myositis is important because of the response to corticosteroids in moderate doses in MCTD, which has been very good.

2.1.5 ANA in the Normal Population

2% of healthy men show ANA with titres of 1 : 10 or more. The incidence is higher in women and some authorities find that 20% of females over the age of 60 are ANA positive. Titres are usually low in healthy people (< 1 : 32).

2.1.6 ANA in SLE

The ANA titres of 95 to 100% of SLE patients are usually 1 : 40 or above although very high titres have been recorded in active disease. Titres are a poor indication of disease activity as they fall only slowly with treatment. All four types of ANA pattern are seen in SLE but the peripheral pattern caused by antibodies to DNA is virtually specific for this disease.

2.1.7 ANA in Liver Disease

There are a number of disorders included in the title chronic active hepatitis (CAH). ANA are common in this group, particularly in the form termed lupoid hepatitis, where titres in excess of 1 : 2000 are sometimes found. In other patients with CAH the ANA tests may be negative or of low titre. The LE cell test may be positive in some patients and occasionally is positive when ANA tests are negative.

ANA occur in about 25% of patients with primary biliary cirrhosis and with alcoholic or cryptogenic cirrhosis. ANA is usually positive in that small group of primary biliary cirrhosis patients who do not have anti-mitochondrial antibodies (Hadziyonnis et al., 1970).

2.1.8 Drug-Induced Lupus

A number of drugs induce a lupus-like illness in a proportion of patients. Such drugs include hydrallazine, procainamide, isoniazid, penicillamine, some anticonvulsants, and chlorpromazine. Documentation is inadequate for the following drugs which have occasionally been suspected of inducing lupus: sulphonamides, penicillin, phenylbutazone, tetracycline, streptomycin, para-aminosalicylic acid, thiouracils, quinidine and griseofulvin.

ANA are present in the great majority of drug-induced lupus cases though the titre is usually low. In contrast with the situation in SLE, complement levels are usually normal and the condition settles on discontinuation of the drug.

The incidence of antinuclear antibodies in various diseases and in control populations is shown in table I.

2.2 Antibodies to Thyroid Antigens

There are a number of different autoantibodies which are associated with diseases of the thyroid gland (Beall and Solomon, 1973). The most important are those directed against:

1) Thyroglobulin
2) Thyroid microsomes
3) Colloid (CA2).

Thyroglobulin and CA2 antigen-antibody systems have been located in the colloid of the thyroid, and the thyroid microsomal system has been shown by ultra-

Table I. The incidence of antinuclear antibodies (ANA) in different disease groups and in control populations (adapted from Pusch [1974] with permission of the author)

Group	Percent with ANA
Connective tissue disorders	
Systemic lupus erythematosus	95-100
Progressive systemic sclerosis	75-80
Rheumatoid arthritis	20-50
Juvenile arthritis	15-30
Felty's syndrome	50
Sjogren's syndrome	85
Chronic discoid lupus erythematosus	35
Dermatomyositis, polymyositis	10-30
Polyarteritis nodosa	30
Suspected connective tissue disease	50
Miscellaneous diseases	
Cirrhosis of the liver	5-20
Post-hepatic cirrhosis	40
Lupoid hepatitis	100
Ulcerative colitis	75
Infective mononucleosis	65
Chronic lymphatic leukaemia	20
Acute leukaemia, lymphatic, myelogenous	25
Waldenstrom's macroglobulinaemia	10-20
Hypergammaglobulinaemic purpura	65
Drug reactions	
Procainamide	50
Hydrallazine	27-50
Isoniazid	20
Chlorpromazine	10-30
Methyldopa	10-20
Chlorthalidone	5-20
Anticonvulsants	30-70
Controls	
Normals	0-4
Healthy 1° relative of SLE patient	0-30
2° relative of SLE patient	0-20
Patients with biological false tests for syphilis	40

centrifugation studies to occur in thyroid epithelial cytoplasm intimately associated with the lipoprotein membrane of the microsomal vesicles.

2.2.1 Assay Techniques

Both immunofluorescent and haemagglutination techniques have been used for detecting thyroglobulin autoantibodies and antibodies to the microsomal antigen but immunofluorescence is the only technique available for detecting CA2. In general, the intensity of staining by immunofluorescence and the strength of the various quantitative results reflect the severity of the thyroid disease and the highest titres occur with thyroiditis.

Two further autoantibodies are demonstrable by bioassay. They are:

1) LATS (Long acting thyroid stimulator, murine thyroid stimulator)

2) LATS-P (LATS protector, human thyroid stimulator).

2.2.2 Thyroid Antibodies in the Normal Population

Thyroid antibodies in low titre are found in some normal subjects and it has been suggested that this reflects the known frequency of focal thyroiditis in the general population. About 1 to 2% of men have antithyroglobulin or antimicrosomal antibodies. The incidence is higher in women (3 to 5%) and increases with age (Bullock et al., 1979). There is little difference in the incidence of thyroglobulin antibodies in men and women over 70 years of age.

Antibody titres < 1 : 400 can be found in patients with normal thyroid function. Most patients with titres above 1 : 800 show abnormalities in thyroid function tests (Wilson, personal communication).

CA2 colloid antibodies can be detected relatively commonly with very sensitive techniques but when sera are screened at a titre of 1 : 10 they are present in less than 1% of normal subjects.

2.2.3 Antithyroid Antibodies in Thyroid Disease (Doniach and Roitt, 1975)

1) Negative tests almost always exclude primary myxoedema. Up to 98% of primary myxoedema patients have antithyroid antibodies, although the incidence of antibodies appear to decrease in long-standing cases.

2) If the tests for thyroid, colloid and cytoplasm antibodies are negative a diagnosis of Hashimoto's thyroiditis can usually be ruled out. These tests are most useful in distinguishing this disease from thyroid cancer and non-toxic goitres. Positive tests are not sufficient to diagnose Hashimoto's disease because antibodies are usually found in other thyroid diseases, especially thyrotoxicosis. Quantitative tests using haemagglutination are used to test these sera.

3) Microsomal or colloid antibodies are found in 85% of thyrotoxic patients and a positive antibody test helps differentiate between mild thyrotoxicosis and anxiety states.

4) CA2 antibodies are present in about 60% of cases of subacute (de Quervain's) thyroiditis.

Table II. Incidence of antithyroid antibodies in thyroid disease and the normal population

Group	Percentage with antibodies			
	Thyroglobulin	Microsomes	CA2	Any of the 3
Hashimoto's thyroiditis	50-90	80-100	50-80	90-100
Thyrotoxicosis	30-60	80-90	> 50	80-90
Primary hypothyroidism	50-60	80-90	50-80	90-98
Non-toxic nodular goitre	0-20 (low titre)	0-10	5-15	< 20 (low titre)
Thyroid carcinoma	0-10 (low titre)	0-10	0-10	< 10 (low titre)
Healthy females	1-5	2-4	4	< 10 (low titre)
Healthy males	1-2	2-3	2	< 5 (low titre)

2.2.4 Antithyroid Antibodies in Other Diseases

1) 50% of pernicious anaemia patients have thyroid antibodies and associated hypothyroidism is common in this disease.

2) Diabetic subjects show an increased incidence of antibodies to thyroid cytoplasm and to gastric parietal cell cytoplasm, irrespective of age and sex.

3) Patients with chronic leprosy have been reported as having an increased incidence of positive thyroglobulin antibodies.

The incidence of antithyroid antibodies in patients with thyroid disease is summarised in table II.

2.3 Gastric Antibodies

Autoantibodies have been reported in patients with chronic atrophic gastritis and pernicious anaemia. These autoantibodies are of two kinds:

a) Autoantibodies to the microsomes of parietal cells of stomach (PCA) have been detected by immunfluorescence using human, pig, or rat stomach as substrate. With rat stomach a much higher proportion of the population shows a positive result (10%).

b) Autoantibodies to the secreted mucoprotein of parietal cell intrinsic factor are detected by radioimmunoassay. There are two antibodies, one inhibiting the binding of vitamin B_{12} to intrinsic factor and one that binds to the preformed intrinsic factor-B_{12} complex.

2.3.1 PCA in Normal Population

Parietal cell antibodies are rarely detected in normal subjects under 30 years of age. A study of the New Zealand normal population by one of the author's group showed an average of 3.1% PCA positive females and 2.1% positive males. About 6% of females and about 2% of males over 30 have PCA. After the age of 60 the figures increase gradually, 15% of females and 12% of males over 70 having PCA (Bullock et al., 1979).

2.3.2 PCA in Disease States

PCA are present in 80 to 90% of patients with pernicious anaemia. In hypochromic anaemias PCA are sometimes found if there is associated atrophic gastritis. In atrophic gastritis without anaemia over 60% of female cases have PCA. There is a smaller incidence in men. About 20% of patients with gastric carcinoma are PCA positive. One-third of thyroiditis and Grave's disease patients have antibodies to gastric parietal cells. The autoantibody has been found to be in the serum of patients with subacute combined degeneration of the spinal cord without other evidence of pernicious anaemia.

The prevalence of PCA in patients with various disorders is shown in table III.

2.3.3 Antibody to Intrinsic Factor

Intrinsic factor antibodies are detected in 55 to 60% of patients with pernicious anaemia but in very few healthy people (Chanarin, 1975).

2.4 Smooth Muscle Antibody (SMA)

This antibody was first reported in patients with chronic active hepatitis and has since been found to be associated with other chronic liver disease (Johnson et al., 1971). It can also can appear transiently in viral infections, such as viral hepatitis and mumps. SMA are identified by immunofluroescence and the results are expressed as a titre.

2.4.1 SMA in the Normal Population

About 2% of the normal population have SMA but some of these cases may be related to recent viral infections (Bullock et al., 1979).

2.4.2 SMA in Liver Diseases

80 to 90% of patients with chronic active hepatitis develop SMA, usually in association with positive ANA and raised IgG. Originally this antibody was thought

Table III. Prevalence of autoantibodies to gastric parietal cells as detected by immunofluorescence, in various disease groups and in the normal population

Group	Percentage positive
Pernicious anaemia	80-90
Atrophic gastritis (females)	60
Atrophic gastritis (males)	Lower incidence than females
Thyroiditis	33
Graves' disease	33
Iron deficiency anaemia	30
Diabetes mellitus	12
Rheumatoid arthritis	5-11
Hashimoto's and primary hypoparathyroidism	30
Normal subjects under 20	0-1
Females 30-70	6
Females over 70	15
Males over 70	12

to be a marker exclusive for chronic active hepatitis and it is true to say that titres of 1 : 80 or greater are rarely found in other disorders; however, between 10 to 50% of patients with primary biliary cirrhosis have SMA, usually in low titres, and about 60% of patients with viral hepatitis develop SMA temporarily.

2.4.3 SMA in Other Diseases

SMA will occur transiently in many viral illnesses. In infectious mononucleosis 80% of patients develop SMA which disappear on recovery (Sutton et al., 1974). This antibody has also been detected in primary atypical pneumonia, upper respiratory infections and in about 10% of patients with rheumatoid arthritis. SMA has also been reported in patients with various forms of cancer.

2.5 Antimitochondrial Antibodies (AMA)

The estimation of these antibodies is particularly useful in the diagnosis of causes of jaundice and liver diseases; they also appear in association with a number of other autoimmune disease but titres are usually low. As they rarely occur in healthy people their presence is a valuable marker. AMA are detected by immunofluorescence using human thyroid, stomach and kidney tissue as substrate.

2.5.1 AMA in the Normal Population

Very few normal people appear to have AMA (0.1 to 0.2%) [Bullock et al., 1979].

2.5.2 AMA in Liver Disease

90% of patients with primary biliary cirrhosis have AMA and about half of these have titres of over 1 : 200 (Sherlock and Scheuer, 1973). In the remainder the titres are moderate or low. There is no correlation with the duration or stage of the disease and the titres tend to remain unchanged on follow-up. Among the few patients with primary biliary cirrhosis who have no AMA about half show ANA or SMA at high titre.

The incidence of AMA varies greatly in chronic active hepatitis and cryptogenic cirrhosis, according to diagnostic criteria. It is rare to find AMA in other forms of cirrhosis, in extrahepatic biliary obstruction or infectious hepatitis.

2.5.3 AMA and Other Diseases

AMA in low titre are found in thyrotoxicosis, Hashimoto's thyroiditis and pernicious anaemia. Addison's disease, myasthenia gravis and autoimmune haemolytic anaemia have an incidence of 1.5 to 3%. In collagen disorders the incidence is slightly higher: rheumatoid arthritis 2%, SLE 5%, and Sjogren's syndrome and systemic sclerosis over 8%. AMA are found at relatively low titre in patients with biological false positive tests for syphilis (WR, VDRL positive, FTA, TPHA negative) see page 52.

2.6 Adrenal Gland Antibodies

Antibodies against adrenal cortical cells occur in approximately 50% of patients with idiopathic Addison's disease and are rarely found apart from this condition. These antibodies do not seem to be influenced by age, sex or duration of the disease and it appears that most patients who develop the antibody do so at an early age. The antibodies are tested for by the immunofluorescence technique.

2.7 Salivary Gland Antibodies

These antibodies are commonly found in Sjogren's syndrome, where 50 to 70% of patients show positive results but they are very rare in any other disease state or in healthy persons. They are also tested for by immunofluorescence.

2.8 Reticulin Antibodies

Reticulin antibodies are found in many patients with dermatitis herpetiformis and coeliac disease, but are also found with increased frequency in chronic heroin addicts, in rheumatoid arthritis and Sjogren's syndrome. About 5% of normal individuals appear to have such antibodies. Reticulin antibodies are tested for by immunofluorescent techniques.

References

Beall, G.D. and Soloman, D.H.: Immunological features of thyroid disease. Postgraduate Medicine 54: 181-189 (1973).

Bullock, J.Y.; Booth, R.J. and Wilson, J.D.: Tissue antibodies in a healthy New Zealand population. New Zealand Medical Journal 89: 11-13 (1979).

Chanarin, I.: The stomach in allergic diseases; in Gell, Coombs and Lachman (Eds) Clinical Aspects of Immunology, p.1429 (Blackwell, Oxford 1975).

Doniach, D. and Roitt, I.M.: Thyroid auto-allergic disease; in Gell, Coombs and Lachman (Eds) Clinical Aspects of Immunology p.1355 (Blackwell, Oxford 1975).

Hadziyonnis, S.; Scheuer, D.J.; Feizi, T.; Naccarato, R.; Doniach, D. and Sherlock, S.: Immunological and histological studies in primary cirrhosis. Journal of Clinical Pathology 23: 95-98 (1970).

Hughes, G.R.V. and Lachman, P.J.: Systemic lupus erythematosus; in Gell, Coombs and Lachman (Eds) Clinical Aspects of Immunology, 3rd Edition p.1122 (Blackwell, Oxford 1975).

Johnson, G.D., Holborow, E.J. and Glynn, L.E.: Antibody to smooth muscle in patients with liver disease. Lancet 2: 878-879 (1971).

Pusch, A.L.: Serodiagnostic tests for syphilis and other diseases; in Davidsohn and Henry (Eds) Clinical Diagnosis by Laboratory Methods p.1232-1235 (Saunders, Philadelphia 1974).

Roitt, I.M.: Interaction of antigen and antibody in vitro; in Essential Immunology, p.99-127 (Blackwell, Oxford 1974).

Sharp, G.C.; Irvin, W.S.; Tan, E.M.; Gould, R.G. and Holman, H.R.: Mixed connective tissue disease — an apparently distinct rheumatic disease syndrome associated with a specific antibody to an extractable nuclear antigen (ENA). American Journal of Medicine 54: 148-159 (1972).

Sherlock, S. and Scheuer, P.J.: Current concepts in primary biliary cirrhosis. New England Journal of Medicine 289: 674-678 (1973).

Sutton, R.N.P; Emand, R.T.D.; Thomas, D.B. and Doniach, D.: The occurrence of autoantibodies in infectious mononucleosis. Clinical Experimental Immunology 17: 423-436 (1974).

Further Reading

Tan, E.M.; Northway, J.D. and Dinnas, J.L.: The clinical significance of antinuclear antibodies. Postgraduate Medicine 54: 143-150 (1973).

Whittingham, S. and Mackay, I.R.: Tissue antigens: autoantigens, alloantigens, xenoantigens, and neoantigens. Review Australian and New Zealand Journal of Medicine 7: 172-194 (1977).

Chapter XIII

Rheumatoid Factors

A rheumatoid factor (RF) is an autoantibody which reacts with IgG. The first rheumatoid factor was described by Waaler (1940) and independently by Rose et al. (1948). Both workers showed that sheep erythrocytes coated with rabbit antibody were agglutinated by a high proportion of sera from rheumatoid subjects. It was later shown that the capacity to agglutinate red cells resided in the gammaglobulin fraction of the patients' sera and eventually the rheumatoid factor was shown to be an immunoglobulin. The classic RF demonstrated by standard laboratory tests belongs to the IgM class. Both IgA and IgG rheumatoid factors have now been found, though their determination is still largely restricted to research laboratories. Rheumatoid factors are found in their highest titre in patients with rheumatoid arthritis but are not restricted to that condition. They will occur in a number of other diseases (table I) and, at low titre, in healthy people.

1. Immunological Tests for IgM Rheumatoid Factors

Two assays are in common use, the sheep cell agglutination test (SCAT), which detects RF against rabbit IgG, and the latex test for RF against human IgG (fig. 1). Patients with rheumatoid factors tend to have a spectrum of rheumatoid factors with differing specificity.

1.1 Sheep Cell Agglutination Test (SCAT)

The SCAT test is based on the fact that IgM RF agglutinates, often to a high titre, sheep or human erythrocytes which have been coated with rabbit anti-erythrocyte antibody. This test is used to detect RF of the IgM class. Titres of more than 1 : 32 are considered to have clinical significance.

Table I. Rheumatoid factor in conditions other than rheumatoid arthritis. From Pusch (1974) with permission of the author and editors

Disease	Percent with positive rheumatoid factor	
	LAT[1]	SCAT[2]
Infectious diseases		
Subacute bacterial endocarditis	48	20
Syphilis	13	5
Viral disease	15	15
Infectious hepatitis	24	20
Trypanosomiasis	27	44
Tuberculosis	11	6
Leprosy	24	15
Lung disease		
Bronchitis	62	18
Asthma	17	0
Asbestosis	21	
Silicosis	15	
Idiopathic pulmonary fibrosis	32	46
Miscellaneous		
Sarcoid	17	5
Multiple myeloma	18	4
Cirrhosis of liver	36	16
Sjogren's syndrome	96	74
Renal homograft	84	8
Myocardial infarction	12	20

1 Latex agglutination test.
2 Sheep cell agglutination test.

1.2 Latex Agglutination Test (LAT)

The latex test uses polystyrene particles coated with human IgG and this forms the basis of a convenient and simple slide agglutination test for RF. In the presence of IgM RF, the latex particles aggregate and can be read easily under a light microscope. Because most rheumatoid patients have a number of different rheumatoid factors which react with various parts of the IgG molecule, rheumatoid sera will usually react with both human and rabbit IgG. Titres of more than 1 : 32 are taken to be significant.

1.3 Comparison of Results Obtained with the SCAT and Latex Tests

In many instances there is no concordance between results obtained with the two tests, i.e. patients may have a positive result from one test but not the other. However, in patients with rheumatoid arthritis, correlation between the two tests is much more common than in patients with other conditions. Rheumatoid factors, particularly those detected by the LAT test, are found in between 1 and 5% of the population, depending upon the sensitivity of the test system used. Less than 25% of RF positive subjects found in a random population study will show any clinical evidence of arthritis.

1.4 Immunological Tests for IgG Rheumatoid Factor

Detection of IgG and IgA rheumatoid factors is difficult and remains largely the province of research laboratories.

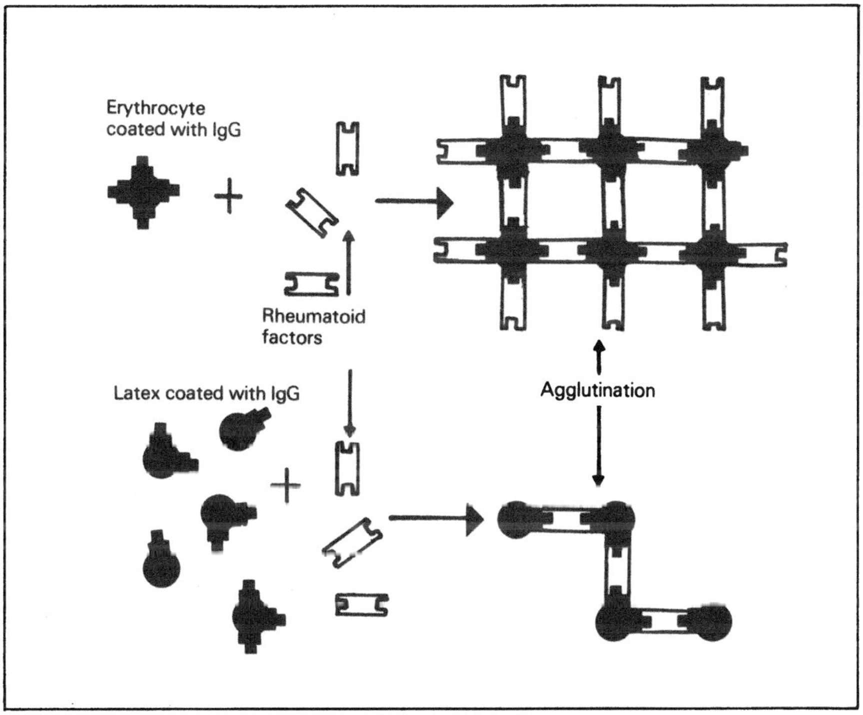

Fig. 1. Principle of sheep cell haemagglutination and latex agglutination reactions in the detection of rheumatoid factor. From Muller (1977) with permission of the author.

2. Clinical Significance of Rheumatoid Factor

2.1 Rheumatoid arthritis

This is a chronic polyarthritis, sometimes with extra-articular manifestations, which affects females more than males, and shows a rising prevalence with age. 70 to 80 % of adult patients with rheumatoid arthritis have RF, usually of high titre, in their serum. The remaining patients have no IgM RF but many, with appropriate tests, may be seen to have IgG or IgA rheumatoid factors. Thus the absence of RF, determined by standard laboratory assays, does not exclude the diagnosis of rheumatoid arthritis. Similarly, the presence of RF cannot be used to make a definite diagnosis.

The role of rheumatoid factors in the pathogenesis of rheumatoid arthritis is unknown. There are a number of disturbances of the immune system seen in this condition and rheumatoid factors and complement may be found deposited in inflamed synovium. It is recognised that those patients with the highest titre rheumatoid factor tend to have a more rapid progression of their arthritis, a poorer prognosis, and more frequently have systemic complications such as nodules, vasculitis, skin ulcers, neuropathy and Felty's syndrome. Additional immunological abnormalities detected in rheumatoid arthritis include a false positive VDRL in up to 10 % of patients, antinuclear antibodies in almost 50 % of patients, and positive LE cells in 10 to 20 %.

2.2 Juvenile Rheumatoid Arthritis

This probably comprises a heterogeneous group of diseases with mono-articular or polyarticular arthropathy in children under the age of 16. About 10 % of patients are found to have IgM rheumatoid factors and this group develop symptoms and signs very similar to adult rheumatoid arthritis. If IgM is purified from the patient's serum before being assayed for RF, the incidence of RF rises to about 40 %. IgG and IgA rheumatoid factors have been identified in some patients with this disease. Complement levels are usually normal or raised as a result of increased synthesis in response to inflammation. About 30 % of affected children have antinuclear antibodies.

2.3 Sjogren's Syndrome

Patients with Sjogren's syndrome have grossly diminished salivary gland and lacrimal secretions with associated drying of the trachea, nose, mouth, eyes and skin. Most of the patients are female and about 50 % have associated rheumatoid arthritis. The incidence of rheumatoid factor is very high in this disease, between 90 and

100 % of patients being positive using the latex test, and about 75 % being positive with the SCAT test. Between 50 and 80 % of the patients have a positive test for antinuclear antibodies and other autoantibodies are found, with lower frequency, particularly antibodies against smooth muscle, thyroid and salivary ducts. A very small proportion of patients may have antibodies to double-stranded DNA. The LE cell phenomena occurs in about 20 % of patients, usually those with associated rheumatoid arthritis.

2.4 Progressive Systemic Sclerosis (Scleroderma)

This condition is characterised by increasing concentrations of collagen in the skin and most organs, and rheumatoid factors are found in about one-third of patients. Antinuclear antibodies, usually of the speckled variety, are present in up to 75 % of patients.

2.5 Systemic Lupus Erythematosus

In this multi-system disease, rheumatoid factors may be detected in up to 50 % of patients.

2.6 Non-arthritic Conditions Associated with Rheumatoid Factor

RFs will occur, sometimes at high titre, in a number of non-rheumatoid conditions. They appear transiently with some bacterial and virus infections, particularly subacute bacterial endocarditis, viral hepatitis and infectious mononucleosis. RFs usually disappear when the inflammatory reaction subsides. They also occur in some chronic and parasitic diseases such as leprosy, schistosomiasis, and fibrosing alveolitis. Some paraproteinaemias have rheumatoid factor-like activity.

In these non-rheumatoid conditions, it is far more common to get a positive result with the latex test than with the SCAT test. However, under some circumstances, both tests are positive.

2.7 Adult Sero-negative Arthritides

IgM rheumatoid factor is not found in ankylosing spondylitis, psoriatic arthritis, or Reiter's disease, yet IgG rheumatoid factors are frequently present in each of these conditions.

In osteoarthritis, gout, rheumatic fever and suppurative arthritis, rheumatoid factors are not found at a greater frequency than is found in the normal population.

References

Muller, W.: Immunological diagnosis of rheumatic diseases. Medical Laboratory 3: 1-14 (1977).

Pusch, A.L.: Serodiagnostic tests for syphilis and other diseases; in Davidsohn and Henry (Eds) Clinical Diagnosis by Laboratory Methods, p.1233 (Saunders, Philadelphia 1974).

Rose, H.M.; Ragan, C.; Pearce, E. and Lipman, M.D.: Differential agglutination of normal and sensitized sheep erythrocytes by sera of patients with rheumatoid arthritis. Proceedings of the Society of Experimental Biology and Medicine 68: 1-6 (1948).

Waaler, E.: On the occurrence of a factor in human serum activating the specific agglutination of sheep blood corpuscles. Acta Pathologica Microbiologica Scandinavica 17: 172 (1940).

Further Reading

Lawrence, J.D.: Rheumatoid factors in families. Seminars in Arthritis and Rheumatism 3: 177-188 (1973).

Waller, M.: Present status of the rheumatoid factor. Critical Reviews in Clinical and Laboratory Science 2: 173-209 (1971).

Walton, K.W.: Hypersensitivity and infection in rheumatic diseases. International Review of Experimental Pathology 6: 285-374 (1968).

Chapter XIV

Skin Tests

In a number of clinical situations *in vitro* laboratory tests are supplemented, or even replaced, by diagnostic skin tests. Here the antigen under investigation is injected into a patient's skin and the subsequent reaction provides diagnostic information. Intradermal injection of antigen can, in sensitised patients, elicit different forms of immune reactions, each with characteristic features. These reactions, and the time intervals between them, are shown in table I. In some circumstances more than one type of reaction can occur concurrently.

Skin tests are used:

a) To identify a patient's response to a specific antigen, as with some bacterial or parasitic infections such as tuberculosis and hydatids
b) To identify inhaled substance such as dust or pollen as the cause of an allergic patient's sensitivity; or one provoking contact dermatitis, by the use of patch skin testing
c) To provide some information regarding the patient's immune status, as with patients who may have immune deficiency diseases, or where the effect on their immune system of malignancy is being evaluated.

1. Mechanism of Skin Reactions

1.1 Immediate Hypersensitivity Reactions (Type I)

This is the classic skin test response for allergic reactions to substances such as dust and pollen. The reaction occurs within 10 to 20 minutes. After foreign antigen penetrates the skin it unites with IgE antibody molecules which are bound to the surface of mast cells in the skin. This provokes the mast cell to 'degranulate' and release a number of vasoactive amines, such as histamine, which produce a local wheal and flare, which is accompanied by itching.

Table I. Skin test reactions

Type of reaction	Interval between skin test and maximal response
Immediate (Type I)	10-20 minutes
Arthus (Type III)	6-20 hours
Delayed (Type IV)	36-72 hours

A further detailed discussion and interpretation of this test is given in chapter XV (page 104).

1.2 Arthus (Type III) Reaction

This response to injected antigen is slower than the Type I reaction and develops some hours after testing, being maximal at about 7 to 8 hours and persisting for 24 to 36 hours. The predominant feature at the reaction site is a soft, widespread oedematous swelling which sometimes has an associated flare. The classic Arthus reaction is produced by the union of circulating IgG antibodies with antigen at the injection site. The immune complexes which form are complement-dependent and produce an intense local reaction. This type of response is of particular interest in some hypersensitivity states, such as farmer's lung. Many patients with asthma and rhinitis who have severe immediate Type I reactions also develop a more delayed reaction which resembles the classic Arthus reaction. There is, however, still some dispute concerning its precise mechanism.

1.3 Delayed Hypersensitivity (Type IV) Reaction

Some antigens, such as proteins extracted from *Mycobacterium tuberculosis,* produce a response in the skin which is largely independent of antibodies and is mediated by T lymphocytes and macrophages. The response takes up to 48 hours to develop and appears as a raised indurated area accompanied by intense itching. Patch tests for substances producing contact dermatitis depend on this reaction where the offending substances unite with proteins in the skin, are then recognised as foreign, and a delayed hypersensitivity reaction occurs.

1.4 Granulomatous Skin Test Reactions

Some skin test materials will produce a reaction that takes some weeks to appear fully, with the development of a granuloma at the injection site. A classical example of this is the Kveim test for sarcoidosis (Siltzbach, 1961).

2. Clinical Application of Skin Tests

2.1 Immediate hypersensitivity (Type I Reaction)

This is discussed in chapter XV (page 105).

2.2 Arthus (Type III) Reaction

This response is used in the diagnosis of the range of conditions termed extrinsic allergic alveolitis. Patients with this pulmonary hypersensitivity state are responding against inhaled substances such as avian antigens in bird-fancier's lung, snuff in pituitary snufftaker's lung, and aspergillis in the condition of allergic bronchopulmonary aspergillosis. In each of these conditions the patients may have precipitin antibodies against the offending substance in their blood. Most will also present a clear Arthus type of reaction to the intradermal injection of these substances. Usually, this reaction is preceded by an immediate Type I reaction which disappears and is followed some hours later by the more prolonged Arthus reaction. In general, these assays are used to provide supporting evidence, as most of the diagnostic information comes from the *in vitro* precipitin antibody test.

2.3 Delayed Hypersensitivity (Type IV Reaction) Skin Tests

There are two major roles for these tests:

a) Diagnosis of a specific disease, e.g. tuberculosis, with the Mantoux reaction
b) General assessment of the patient's cell-mediated immunity, e.g. as a prognostic aid in cancer, particularly lymphomas, or in assessing someone for immune deficiency.

2.3.1 Diagnosis of Specific Diseases

Tuberculosis. The Mantoux reaction is the most widely employed of the specific delayed hypersensitivity skin tests. Two forms of antigen are used, both of which are prepared from the *Mycobacterium tuberculosis:*

a) Old tuberculin which is simply an autoclaved culture filtrate of *M. tuberculosis*. An international standard is available against which commercial extracts are compared.
b) Purified protein derivative (PPD) which is an ammonium sulphate precipitate from the *M. tuberculosis* culture filtrate. This is the preparation most widely used.

Two techniques are in common use to apply the antigen — they use either intradermal injection (Mantoux) or the Heaf gun, which is a multipuncture gun with

6 needles which can be set to penetrate the skin to 1 to 2mms. Reactions are measured by the diameter of the wheal and those greater than 5mm are taken as positive.

10 units of PPD is a standard test dose. Patients with active TB may react vigorously with this dose and can even produce very strong reactions to one unit. In contrast, healthy people who have had no, or insignificant, contact with the disease, or have not received a BCG vaccination, usually give a negative response to up to 100 units.

Reactions to PPD will become positive as early as 4 to 5 days after BCG vaccination, so should be positive in most patients presenting with active tuberculosis. However, a small proportion of patients, usually those with most active infections such as miliary tuberculosis, will have negative reactions. The mechanism for this is not entirely understood but may depend on an interaction between anti-TB antibody and effector T cells for delayed hypersensitivity reaction. In this circumstance a positive *in vitro* reaction can often be obtained with the patient's lymphocytes mixed with PPD, producing transformation and division of the lymphocytes *in vitro* (See chapter XVI — Lymphocyte Function Tests).

Leprosy: The lepromin test uses extracts of lepromatous skin nodules which are sterilised and ground up for injection. The reaction is a classic Type IV reaction reaching a peak at 48 hours. A later reaction usually develops slowly, appearing at 7 days and lasting for up to 4 weeks. The majority of patients with the tuberculoid form of leprosy will react, whereas those with the lepromatous form usually give a negative response.

Hydatids: The Casoni test uses extracts of *Echinococcus granulosa* cysts which have been chemically purified and lyophilised (Kagan et al., 1966). Patients with present or past hydatids will respond. The reaction has two phases: first a wheal develops, which reaches a maximum in 15 minutes, and this represents a classic Type I hypersensitivity reaction; within about 24 hours a later reaction develops, with oedema at the injection site but little erythema. This has many of the features of an Arthus reaction.

Candida: Patients with current or past candida infections usually have a strong delayed hypersensitivity reaction to candida antigen injected intradermally. The diagnosis of candida infections is usually made visually or by culture of the organism, and the skin test reaction is aimed more at investigating the patient's immune reactivity. The disorder of mucocutaneous candidiasis is very uncommon and although these patients present with chronic candida infections, usually of the nails and mouth, they lack a positive skin test to candida.

Contact dermatitis: The potential agents suspected of provoking an individual patient's dermatitis are placed on small test strips on a patient's skin. They are left in place for up to 48 hours and are then read. A number of tiny raised indurated areas indicate a positive response. As with other delayed hypersensitivity tests, the reaction will be inhibited by systemic steroids.

Table II. Conditions associated with depressed delayed hypersensitivity

Congenital immune deficiency
Combined non-classifiable immune deficiency
Thymic aplasia
Ataxia telangiectasia
Nezclof's syndrome
Mucocutaneous candidiasis
Infections or immunisation
Mumps
Infectious mononucleosis
Rubella
Influenza
Hepatitis B
Tuberculosis
Lepromatous leprosy
Malignant tumours
Hodgkin's disease
Non-Hodgkin's lymphoma
Acute leukaemia
Carcinoma colon
Other conditions
Sarcoidosis
Uraemia
Cirrhosis of the liver

2.3.2 General Assessment of Cell-Mediated Immunity

There are three reasons for using these skin tests to assess a patient's immune system. Firstly, as part of a workup for patients with malignant disease, particularly Hodgkin's disease; absent delayed hypersensitivity reactions are associated with more extensive disease while recovery of these reactions following therapy is a good prognostic sign. Secondly, to investigate potential cases of immune deficiency. Thirdly, as a prognostic aid following trauma where the loss of reactivity to injected antigens is a very poor prognostic sign.

There are two ways of assessing patient's cell-mediated immunity. First, by using a battery of commonly encountered antigens, to at least one of which most healthy people should be able to respond. A commonly used battery includes purified protein derivative (PPD), mumps, *Candida albicans*, trichophyton, and streptokinase-streptodornase (SKSD). About 95% of healthy people will respond to at least one of these and an absence of response frequently has clinical significance. People without responses are termed anergic and the frequency of anergy is greatly increased in patients with malignancy, particularly in those over 50 years. Secondly, where skin tests are negative, the patient can be deliberately sensitised with an agent they would not previously have encountered, and then re-checked for their capacity to mount a reaction. The substance most commonly used is dinitrochlorobenzene (DNCB) which is applied to the skin, the patient then being re-challenged after 10 days.

2.3.3 Diminished or Absent Delayed Hypersensitivity Responses

Conditions where a generalised depression of the patient's cell-mediated immunity occurs are listed in table II. Some viruses are potent immunosuppressive agents. Following measles, patients may lose their capacity to mount a Mantoux reaction for anything between 4 and 8 weeks.

References

Kagan, I.G.; Osiman, J.J.; Varela, J.C. and Allain, D.S.: Evaluation of intradermal and serologic tests for the diagnosis of hydatid disease. American Journal of Tropical Medicine 15: 172-183 (1966).

Siltzbach, L.E.: The Kveim test in sarcoidosis: a study of 750 patients. Journal of the American Medical Association 178: 476-483 (1961).

Further Reading

Pepys, J.: Skin testing. British Journal of Hospital Medicine 14: 412-417 (1975).

Chapter XV

Allergy Tests

Several common conditions are recognised as having an allergic aetiology, e.g. rhinitis (seasonal and perennial), urticaria, asthma, contact dermatitis, anaphylaxis and sometimes eczema (atopic dermatitis). The term allergic aetiology implies that the patient reacts to some specific external agent and the tissue damage or inflammation resulting from that interaction is revealed by particular symptoms, e.g. hayfever with pollens. It is now recognised that in some of the disease groups listed above, some patients have clear allergic precipitating factors, while others do not, e.g. extrinsic and intrinsic asthma, allergic and vasomotor rhinitis.

A variety of tests are available which provide evidence of a patient's allergic status, i.e. whether they are atopic or not (roughly meaning having an allergic constitution) and tests can be used to identify particular substances or allergens provoking the patient's symptoms. It is important to define the allergic basis of a patient's disorder as management is frequently dictated by the result. In some instances it is possible to avoid the allergen and this is obviously mandatory, where possible, in patients who have had an anaphylactic reaction. In some circumstances desensitisation to individual allergens may provide control of the patient's symptoms.

1. Mechanisms of Allergic Reactions

The discovery of IgE as the reaginic antibody which mediates most allergic reactions put the aetiology of allergy on a much sounder theoretical basis (Ishizaka and Ishizaka, 1975). However, it should be remembered that not all so-called allergic reactions are IgE-mediated.

When allergen interacts with IgE attached to mast cells, symptoms will appear in 10 to 20 minutes. IgG may be involved in some types of asthma when the reaction between antibody and allergen is followed by symptoms of bronchospasm after some hours. In contact dermatitis the allergic mechanism is mediated by T lymphocytes and macrophages and not by antibody at all. It is also possible that some reactions to foods may involve non-immunological mechanisms, as in chocolate or red wine-induced migraine.

2. Diagnosis of Atopy

If patients with asthma, rhinitis and urticaria can be shown to have an allergic tendency, i.e. are atopic, a search should be made for the offending allergens. A diagnosis of atopy depends on one or more of the following pieces of evidence:

1) The patient's symptoms are clearly produced by an external allergen
2) Positive reaction to either bronchial or nasal provocation
3) There is a strong family history of allergy
4) The presence of eosinophilia (which is not diagnostic alone, but good supportive evidence), or presence of many eosinophils in nasal or bronchial secretions
5) Raised IgE levels (although, as with eosinophilia, these can occur with some parasitic infections)
6) Positive immediate hypersensitivity skin tests
7) Positive RAST test to likely allergens.

Some asthmatic patients without a family history of allergy and with negative skin tests still can be shown to have allergen-induced asthma, sometimes from substances to which they are exposed in their occupations.

3. Tests for Allergy

The following tests are those in common use in the management of allergic problems. The use of a number of other procedures, such as provocation testing, is restricted to specialist centres and will be only cursorily mentioned. Tests such as subcutaneous provocation and the leukocyte cytotoxicity test remain to be clearly established as aids in the diagnosis of allergy.

3.1 Eosinophilia

3.1.1 Peripheral Blood Eosinophils

A raised percentage of eosinophils in the peripheral blood leukocytes has long been recognised as a feature in atopic patients. A more reliable index than percentage is the total eosinophil count per mm^3 or x 10^9/litre. Excluding atopic people, the mean total eosinophil count (TEC) for a healthy population is 0.1×10^9/litre ($100/mm^3$) and rarely exceeds 0.25×10^9/litre ($250/mm^3$).

In patients with bronchial asthma, whether extrinsic or intrinsic, TEC levels usually exceed 0.35 x 10^9/litre (350/mm^3).

Lowell (1975) has suggested that the total eosinophil count is of value in monitoring corticosteroid therapy in bronchial asthma, a fall of total eosinophil count to the normal range usually preceding a good clinical response. He also suggested that the presence of eosinophilia in asthmatic patients with obstructive pulmonary manifestations indicates a significant reversible element of airways obstruction.

It is important to remember eosinophilia occurs in many conditions other than atopy and is certainly present in many patients with intrinsic rather than extrinsic asthma. Its presence, however, provides some evidence of atopy.

3.1.2 Eosinophils in Nasal and Bronchial Washings

Sputum and nasal swabs are spread on a slide, fixed for 5 minutes in ethanol and then stained with Hansel's stain for eosinophils. A nasal smear is best taken by inserting a swab into the nose, leaving it in place for 2 minutes, to stimulate rhinorrhoea, and then smearing the swab on a slide. An alternative technique is to smear beneath the inferior turbinate. In people with allergic rhinitis or extrinsic asthma, the mucous secretions contain a predominance of eosinophils. Although not definitive, the finding of large numbers of eosinophils in either situation is strong presumptive evidence of an allergic process.

3.2 Serum Immunoglobulins

3.2.1 IgA

IgA is readily measured by immunodiffusion. Normal values are 1.5 to 4.0g/litre. It is now well recognised that patients with immunodeficiency diseases have a significantly increased incidence of allergic conditions. In atopic patients immune deficiency, especially of IgA, occurs more frequently than in non-atopics. It therefore seems important in children presenting with allergic manifestations, particularly where they are experiencing recurrent infections, that serum immunoglobulins be estimated for evidence of congenital immunoglobulin deficiencies. Selective IgA deficiency is the commonest of the immunoglobulin deficiency disorders.

3.2.2 IgE

IgE is determined by a radioimmunoassay. The method is accurate and the results are expressed in international units of IgE/ml with a normal range up to 150 iu/ml in healthy adults. At birth infants have almost no IgE in their serum. Adult levels are reached by the age of 4 to 5 years. Mean IgE levels are about 9iu/ml by 5 months and 30iu/ml by the age of 1 year (Kjellman et al., 1976). Atopic subjects in general have significantly higher IgE levels than healthy subjects. In general, the highest IgE levels are observed in patients with evidence of reactivity to a large number of allergens. About 60% of asthmatic patients have raised IgE levels and these levels may rise on exposure to allergens, for instance during the pollen season.

IgE levels in allergic disorders: IgE levels are elevated in 60 to 70% of patients with extrinsic asthma but in only 5% of patients with intrinsic asthma (Pepys and Davies, 1977).

Elevated IgE levels are also observed among patients with atopic eczema, allergic rhinitis and conjunctivitis and those with bronchopulmonary aspergillosis.

However, the majority of patients with allergic rhinitis and conjunctivitis have levels in the normal range although the mean IgE level for this group is 3 times the normal mean for age. IgE levels increase with heavy exposure to allergen and, temporarily, early in a desensitisation course and may persist as markedly elevated levels long after clinical symptoms have subsided.

IgE levels in non-allergic disorders: IgE levels may become elevated as the result of non-allergic disorders (Johansson et al., 1972). Elevated levels have been reported in many parasitic diseases, bullous pemphigus and thymic aplasia. Levels are markedly elevated in Job's syndrome and Wiskott-Aldrich syndrome, and moderately but significantly elevated in patients with the Di-George syndrome, some forms of combined immunodeficiency syndrome and Hodgkin's disease.

IgE in diagnosis: Allergy has been shown to develop during the first year of life in 83% of infants with IgE levels between 20 and 100iu/ml (Kjellman and Johannson, 1976). Serum IgE levels may be useful in determining which patients should undergo skin testing or other forms of evaluation for allergies.

Positive skin tests for immediate hypersensitivity are rarely found in infants and young children with IgE levels in the low or normal range and are uncommon among children and adults with IgE levels < 100iu/ml. Positive tests occur in most patients with IgE levels above 100iu/ml.

3.3 Skin Tests

A variety of different reactions can occur in sensitised patients after antigen is injected into their skin. These are discussed in chapter XIV (page 95). Details of the immediate hypersensitivity tests used to identify allergens in most patients with allergy are described below.

3.3.1 Skin Test Techniques

Type 1 hypersensitivity reactions are detected by one of three methods. The most satisfactory is the *prick test* where a row of test substances is placed on the patient's arm or back. The skin is pricked through each droplet with a small blood lancet which is wiped between each droplet to avoid a carryover of test substances. When tests are carried out on the forearm reactivity decreases in proportion to the distance

Table I. Drugs and immediate hypersensitivity skin reactions

Inhibitors of reaction
Antihistamines — potent
Isoproterenol (sublingual only) — weak
Adrenaline (subcutaneous) — transient
Drugs without effect
Corticosteroids
Aminophylline
Ephedrine
Sodium cromoglycate

from the cubital fossa and is less on the radial than ulnar side. A strong positive reaction is a wheal greater than 5mm diameter.

The *scratch test* depends on placing a series of superficial scratches on the patient's skin and the test material is applied to the scratch. Results are more variable than with the prick test.

Intradermal injections of 0.02 to 0.05ml of test substance can be used but this method is very sensitive and cumbersome.

3.3.2 Inhibitors of Skin Test Reactions

It should be emphasised that some drugs, particularly antihistamines, are potent inhibitors of this reaction and should be discontinued for at least 48 hours before skin testing (table I).

Sympathomimetics of older type such as adrenaline or isoprenaline may produce short term cutaneous vasoconstriction and thus prevent the dilation necessary for positive skin response.

Patients who have suffered an anaphylactic reaction should not be tested within 2 weeks of the reaction as skin test reactivity is depressed.

3.3.3 Interpretation of a Positive Skin Test

Some substances are sufficiently irritant to produce a positive reaction in many or most of the people tested. Therefore the concentration of test substance has to be sufficiently low as to ensure that in most people tested positive reactions indicate a specific immune response.

Dermatographism may give false positives in 5 to 20% of patients and because almost all tests will be positive in these subjects, their degree of positivity should be related to a control glycerine-saline test done at the same time.

It is very important to remember that a positive skin test does not necessarily indicate clinical sensitivity to that test substance. IgE is not always fixed to both the skin and to target organs such as the nose, in individual patients. Many people with widespread skin reactivity to many allergens may have no clinical symptoms. The positive test should be interpreted very carefully in the light of the patient's history and act as a guide to the allergen involved rather than as a proven fact.

Positive skin test reactivity to foods has limited value as there is probably only a 20% correlation between clinical sensitivity to certain foods and positive skin tests. It should be remembered that some patients have allergies to the digestive products of foods and not to the food as initially presented.

Negative skin tests may occur because the patient has no allergies to the test substance. However, they occur also because the skin test preparations are too weak and some allergy extracts lose potency on storage. It is important to know that the individual extracts being used are effective enough to produce good reactions. The skin test substance has to penetrate deeply enough to provoke a reaction and with the prick test a too superficial penetration may limit positivity. In very young infants and in very old people the incidence of positivity is much less and the reactivity of skin in these circumstances is low. The incorporation of a histamine control in the test battery will give an index of the patient's innate skin reactivity. Finally, as previously mentioned, certain drugs will inhibit skin test reaction and should be avoided.

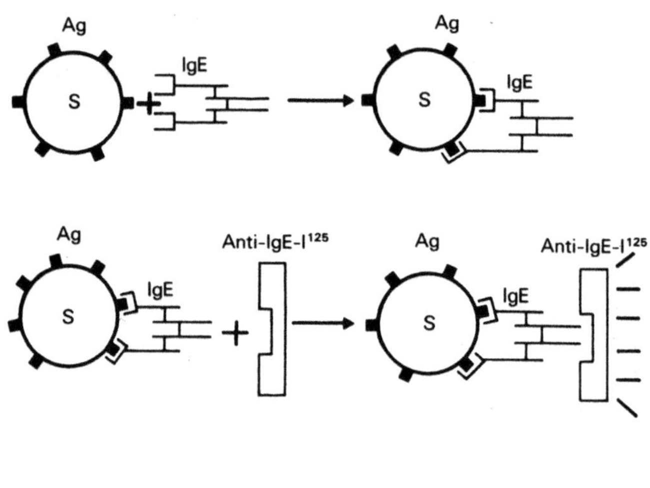

Fig. 1. The RAST test. The sorbent S has antigenic determinants to which human IgE becomes attached and is detected by labelling with radiolabelled anti IgE. Adapted from Frick (1978) with permission of the author and editors.

3.4 Radioallergosorbent Test (RAST)

The immediate hypersensitivity reaction depends upon union between an allergen and a specific antiallergenic IgE molecule. An *in vitro* test has been developed to identify specific IgE against allergens. In this RAST assay patient's serum is incubated with selected substances coupled to cellulose discs (Wide et al., 1967). If a specific IgE is present, it binds the allergen and is then detected by a radio-labelled anti-IgE antiserum (fig. 1). This test is reliable and accurate and in general correlates very well with both skin test reactivity and provocation tests. Its advantage lies:

1) In patients with severe dermatographism when interpretation of skin tests is difficult
2) In elderly patients with non-reactive skin
3) In patients with severe skin diseases who cannot otherwise be tested
4) In very young children
5) Where an allergen is potentially hazardous to the patient, as with antibodies against bee venom
6) Where an allergy produces positive skin reaction by directly liberating histamine
7) In providing firm clear objective evidence that a patient has raised IgE against an allergen before initiating desensitisation.

The RAST test is expensive and only a limited number of allergens are available. However, it is likely that both skin test material and desensitisation vaccines will be standardised as the basis of RAST positivity and therefore this assay procedure should become a standard assay in laboratories dealing with allergy problems.

References

Frick, O.L.: Immediate hypersensitivity; in Fudenberg, Stites, Caldwell and Wells (Eds) Basic and Clinical Immunology, p.246-266 (Lange Medical Publications, California, 1978).

Ishizaka, T. and Ishizaka, K.: Biology of immunoglobulin E.: molecular basis of reaginic hypersensitivy. Progress in Allergy 19: 60-171 (1975).

Johansson, S.G.O.; Bernich, H. and Berg, T.: The clinical significance of IgE; in Schwartz (Ed) Progress in Clinical Immunology. Vol. 1, p.153 (Grune and Stratton, New York 1973).

Kjellman, N-I.M. and Johansson, S.G.O.: IgE and atopic allergy in newborn and infants with a family history of atopic disease. Acta Paediatrica Scandinavica 65: 601-607 (1976).

Kjellman, N-I.M.; Johansson, S.G.O. and Roth, A.: Serum IgE levels in healthy children quantified by a sandwich technique (PRIST). Clinical Allergy 6: 51-59 (1976).

Lowell, F.C.: The total eosinophil count in obstructive pulmonary disease. New England Journal of Medicine 292: 1182-1183 (1975).

Pepys, J. and Davies, R.J.: Allergy; in Clark and Godfrey (Eds) Asthma, p.51-59 (Chapman and Hall, London 1977).

Wide, L.; Bennich, H. and Johansson, S.G.O.: Diagnosis of allergy by an in-vitro test for allergen antibodies. Lancet 2: 1105-1106 (1967).

Chapter XVI

Lymphocyte Function Tests

Lymphocytes are small cells (8-12μ in diameter) with relatively large nuclei. They have the capacity to circulate throughout the body in both blood and extracellular fluid which is important, as they play a vital role in the defence of the body against infection. Although other cells, such as neutrophils, may be more aggressive in destroying antigens, lymphocytes have a particular function because they are the only cells which have the ability to recognise that an antigen is foreign and not part of the host tissue.

There are several subgroups of lymphocytes and these have different functions. The two major groups are termed T and B lymphocytes and are indistinguishable from each other under the light microscope. All lymphocytes originate from bone marrow stem cells and, by different pathways of differentiation, are distributed during fetal life to peripheral lymphoid tissues such as the spleen, lymph nodes, tonsils and Peyer's patches. T lymphocytes undergo differentiation within the thymus and B lymphocytes within the bone marrow (fig. 1).

1. Subgroups of Lymphocytes

Various lymphocyte subpopulations are identified by way of specialised structures termed receptors on the cell surface. Each subpopulation has a different function. The most important receptors on human lymphocytes are depicted in figure 2.

1.1 Sheep Red Blood Cell (SRBC) Receptor

T lymphocytes have the capacity *in vitro* to bind SRBC to their surface to form a rosette. This phenomenon may have no biological significance but is a useful and accurate marker for the identification of T lymphocytes.

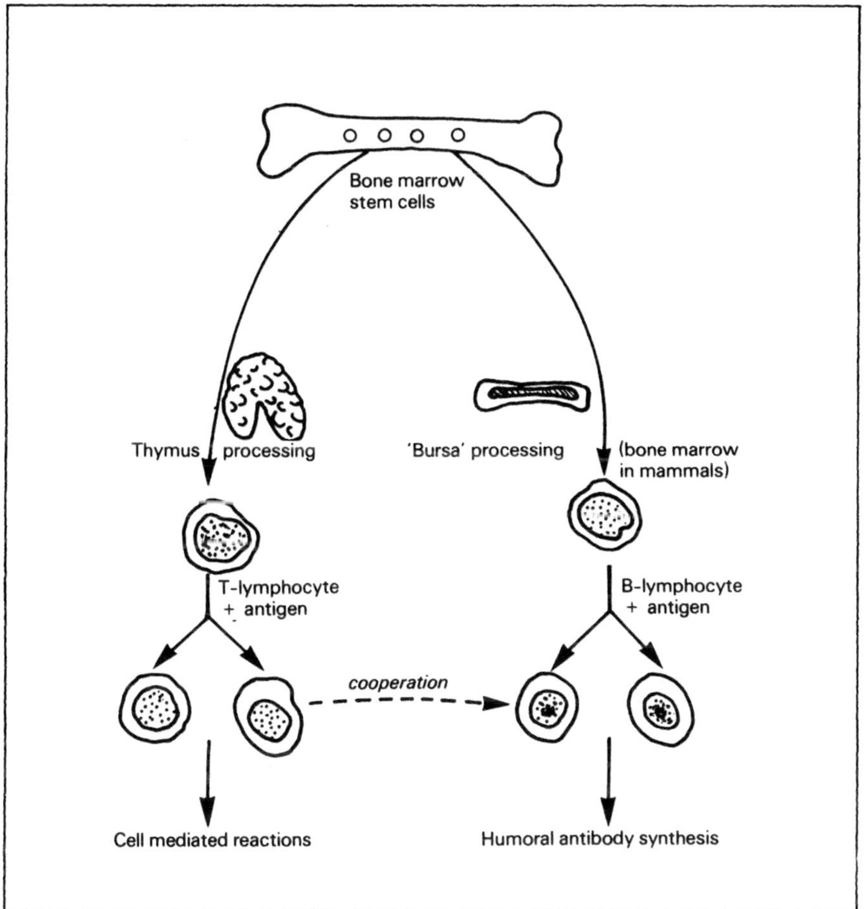

1

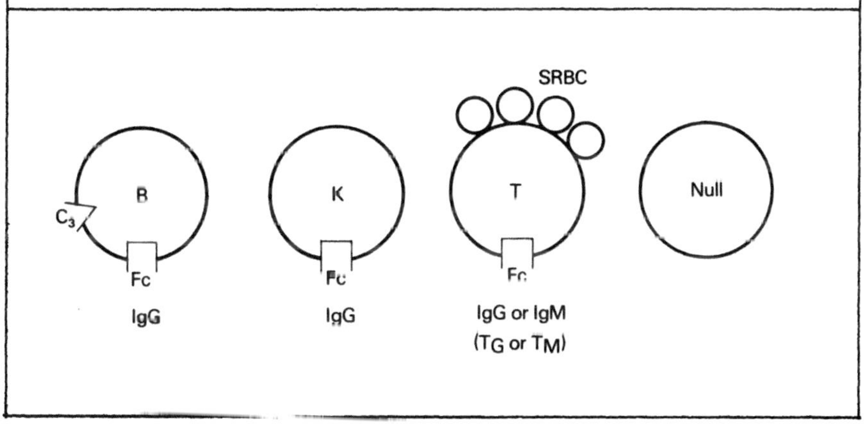

2

Fig. 1. Differentiation of lymphocyte populations.

Fig. 2. Surface receptors on human lymphocyte subgroups.

1.2 Surface Immunoglobulin (SIg)

B lymphocytes synthesise immunoglobulin which then forms an integral part of their cell membrane. They recognise a foreign antigen by way of their cell-bound SIg.

1.3 Fc Receptors

Most lymphocyte subpopulations have the capacity to bind the Fc portion of immunoglobulin molecules to their surface. One population of lymphocytes (K lymphocytes) lacks both SIg and the SRBC receptor. However these cells have very strong (avid) Fc receptors. Weaker Fc receptors are present on B lymphocytes and on T lymphocytes. For most cells the Fc receptors bind IgG_1 and IgG_3. However a small population of T lymphocytes will bind the Fc portion of IgM (T_M). This distinguishes it from other T lymphocytes which have Fc receptors for IgG (T_G) (Moretta et al., 1977).

1.4 Complement Receptors

B lymphocytes have the capacity strongly to bind the third component of complement (C3).

2. Function of Lymphocyte Subpopulations

2.1 T Lymphocytes

There are a number of different T lymphocyte subpopulations which have different functions. Overall, T lymphocytes are necessary for both the recognition and effector arms of cell-mediated immunity which provides defences against fungi and many viruses. A classic example of a T cell reaction is the Mantoux reaction. Other T lymphocytes are necessary to assist B lymphocytes to generate antibody and these are called T helper cells.

These can be recognised as T lymphocytes with Fc receptors for IgM (T_M cells). Other T lymphocytes have the capacity to suppress immunoglobulin production and are recognised by having Fc receptors for IgG (T_G cells). Some T lymphocytes may suppress other T lymphocytes producing cell-mediated immunity.

2.2 B Lymphocytes

These cells synthesise immunoglobulin and develop into plasma cells.

2.3 K Lymphocytes

These cells are effective against foreign cells or bacteria by destroying those cells when they are coated with antibodies. This process is termed 'antibody-dependent cell cytotoxicity' (ADCC).

2.4 Null Cells

A small proportion of lymphocytes appear to carry no receptor. They may be precursors of other lymphocytes or they may be committed lymphocytes which have lost their receptors. In some patients they represent malignant cells.

3. Laboratory Assays

Most tests to identify lymphocyte populations or to evaluate lymphocyte function *in vitro* require lymphocytes to be purified from a peripheral blood sample. This is done by taking blood and spinning it through gradients composed of solutions of selected density. Red cells and neutrophils will be spun through the gradient and lymphocytes and macrophages are separated onto the top of the gradient solution. By this means, a relatively pure population of lymphocytes can be obtained simply for assays described below.

3.1 Identification of Lymphocyte Receptors

3.1.1 SRBC Receptor

Purified lymphocytes are mixed *in vitro* with sheep red blood cells, firstly at 37° and then at 4°C for up to 2 hours. The cells are then gently resuspended and examined under a counting chamber where T lymphocytes will be seen surrounded by a halo of SRBC forming a rosette. B, K, null cells and macrophages will not bind the sheep red blood cells under these circumstances.

3.1.2. Surface Immunoglobulin

Fluorescein-labelled anti-human immunoglobulin is incubated with purified lymphocytes which are then examined under a fluorescent microscope. The cells with surface immunoglobulin will be seen to fluoresce while T lymphocytes will not. Lymphocytes with strong Fc receptors, such as K lymphocytes, may well have bound *in vivo* sufficient IgG to be seen as fluorescing cells by this method. Pre-incubation of the lymphocytes for 30 minutes at 37° will release this passively bound immunoglobulin to reveal the B lymphocytes as the only cells which synthesise their own surface immunoglobulin (Horwitz and Lobo, 1975).

3.1.3 Fc Receptors

These can be identified either by the lymphocyte's capacity to bind IgG passively and then lose it on heating, or by a rosette technique using red cells coated with antibody. These then are mixed with purified lymphocytes, the antibody on the surface of the red cells binds to the Fc receptor and the cells are identified as a rosette.

3.1.4 Complement Receptors

These too are identified by a rosette technique where antibody plus complement are bound to the surface of a red cell and then mixed with the lymphocytes under test.

3.2 Tests of Lymphocyte Function

3.2.1 T Cells

The four most common assays are:

a) Delayed hypersensitivity reactions
b) Phytohaemagglutinin response
c) Specific blast cell transformations
d) Mixed lymphocyte reactions.

Delayed hypersensitivity tests: These are discussed elsewhere (page 96) and are a very effective assay for T cell function as they depend both on recognition of foreign antigen and on the generation of a full effector response.

PHA response: Lymphocytes are mixed *in vitro* with a polysaccharide, phytohaemagglutinin (PHA) extracted from beans. This substance is a mitogen which has the capacity to switch T lymphocytes into cell cycle whereby they synthesise DNA, turn into blast cells and ultimately divide. This capacity to divide when confronted with PHA is measured by culturing the lymphocytes for 3 days and measuring the portion of DNA synthesised by a radio assay.

Specific antigen-induced transformation: A small proportion of T lymphocytes will respond to some antigens added to cultures of lymphocytes *in vitro*. These cells will, over the course of 5 or 6 days, divide sufficiently to be detected by the radio assay for DNA synthesis as used in the PHA response.

Mixed lymphocyte reaction: When lymphocytes from two different people are mixed together in culture, each will recognise the other cells as foreign and undergo blast transformation as a reaction against the foreign antigen. This is a strong reaction and can be measured by the amount of DNA synthesised.

One-way mixed lymphocyte reactions can be produced by inhibiting the division of lymphocytes from one of the lymphocyte populations. This is done by treating these cells either with radiation or by the cytotoxic drug mitomycin-C. By this technique the treated cells are called stimulating cells and the other lymphocytes are the responder population. This assay is a sensitive index of T lymphocyte function and is also used to determine histocompatability differences between the two populations (described in chapter XIX).

3.2.2 Tests of B Cell Function

These include:

a) Immunoglobulin levels (see chapter X)
b) Rise in antibody levels following immunisation
c) Isohaemagglutinin levels
d) *In vitro* immunoglobulin production by lymphocytes stimulated with pokeweed mitogen (PWM).

Immunoglobulin levels: These are described elsewhere (see page 60).

Rise in antibody following immunisation: A patient's reaction to a specific immunisation can give a considerable amount of information about their B cell function. After immunisation antibody levels are measured and the patient is then rechallenged with the immunising agent and the secondary level evaluated.

Isohaemagglutinin levels: Even when normal immunoglobulin levels have been found in patients, there may still be some defect of antibody activity. Measurement of naturally occurring isohaemagglutinins against red cell antigens gives some measure of humoral responses.

In vitro immunoglobulin production by lymphocytes stimulated with pokeweed: This is a sophisticated assay which depends upon stimulating purified lymphocytes in culture with a mitogen, pokeweed (PWM) which stimulates not only T lymphocytes but also some B lymphocytes. The end result of the reaction, over the course of 5 or 6 days, is determined by immunofluorescence when a proportion of peripheral blood cells will have concentrations of immunoglobulin in their cytoplasm.

4. Clinical Interpretation

4.1 Altered Lymphocyte Populations

Various surface markers are of clinical interest because they assist in the understanding of various diseases, especially lymphoproliferative ones.

4.1.1 Chronic Lymphocytic Leukaemia

In this disease there is a proliferation of relatively mature lymphocytes (usually B cells) and more than 70% of a patient's circulating lymphocytes show surface immunoglobulin (Wilson and Nossal, 1971). In about 10 to 20% of cases of chronic lymphocytic leukaemia (CLL) the proliferating cells do not show surface immunoglobulin although it has been suggested that the cells show reduced levels rather than an absence of immunoglobulin. T cell CLL occurs occasionally. In many cases of CLL a serum monoclonal immunoglobulin (commonly IgM) is found. Patients with CLL show an increased tendency to develop other malignancies.

4.1.2 Acute Lymphocytic Leukaemia

This disease is a malignant proliferation of early cells in the lymphoid series and it is found most commonly in children. In several studies approximately 20% of acute lymphocytic leukaemia (ALL) patients have been shown to form sheep erythrocyte rosettes (T cells) [Catovsky et al., 1974]. Most patients' lymphocyte cells lack both surface immunoglobulin and Fc receptors. They are termed null cells but their relationship to the null cells in normal peripheral blood is unknown.

A number of immunological tests can assist in the overall prognosis in ALL children. A poorer prognosis is indicated when there are abnormalities in specific immunity and general immune function. The 20% of patients with T cell acute leukaemia have a higher median age, a poorer response to treatment, and a worse prognosis (Catovsky et al., 1974).

4.1.3 Post-radiation Effect

After radiation there are alterations to the relative numbers of lymphocyte cells. There is an increase in B cells which may last months or years. There is also an increase in the absolute number of K cells with a noticeable increase in the relative percentage of these cells (Wilson et al., unpublished data). In contrast the number of T cells decreases and there is a marked lack of response to the mitogen phytohaemagglutinin. Both these effects may last for a period of months or years.

4.1.4 Post-corticosteroid Effect

Corticosteroids have an immunosuppressive action. A single oral or intravenous pharmacological dose of corticosteroid can significantly change the profile of circulating white blood cells. There is a decrease in the number of circulating lymphocytes, monocytes and eosinophils, but an increase in neutrophils. The changes are at peak about 4 to 6 hours after the dose has been administered and there may be a return to normal within 24 hours. There is a decrease in the absolute number of both B and T lymphocytes but normally T cells are more affected (Wilson et al., 1974).

T cells also show a marked decrease in response to isoantigens, specific antigens and mitogens but these changes are transitory. It has been proposed that some T cell subpopulations may be resistant to corticosteroid inhibition.

The effects of corticosteroids on B cells are much less obvious. IgG catabolism has been shown to be increased by corticosteroid treatment and there is a depression in circulating IgG, not all of which can be attributed to increased catabolism.

4.2 Abnormalities of Lymphocyte Function

Generalised depression of T cell function is detected by changes in PHA responses or in delayed hypersensitivity skin tests (see chapter XIV). Specific defects are evaluated by studying antigen stimulation of lymphocytes in culture, or by specific delayed hypersensitivity skin tests.

4.2.1 Malignant Diseases

Many patients with cancer will show generalised depression of T lymphocyte function. This is most frequently observed in patients over the age of 50 and in those with more extensive tumours. About 50% of patients of all ages with lymphomas, particularly Hodgkin's disease, will show depressed T cell function (Sumner and Wilson, unpublised data). With more sophisticated tests the percentage of abnormal reactions is higher. Recovery of T cell function following therapy is a very good prognostic sign and is often seen in lymphoma patients following chemotherapy. Radiotherapy results in depressed PHA responses for months or years afterwards. In these patients however, recovery of delayed hypersensitivity skin tests is common.

4.2.2 Infectious Diseases

T lymphocytes show depressed activity during and following some infections such as hepatitis B, measles, cytomegalovirus and other viral infections not always identifiable. Usually these changes are transient.

4.2.3 Immune Deficiency

These conditions are discussed fully in chapter XXI. Patients with Di George syndrome and Nezelof's syndrome have absent or weak PHA responses. Patients with chronic mucocutaneous candidiasis will show absent T cell responses to candida *in vitro*, and absent delayed hypersensitivity skin reactions to candida, although reactions to other antigens are usually intact.T lymphocyte defects are associated with immunoglobulin deficiencies and are fully described in chapter XXI.

4.2.4 Sarcoidosis

Mild to moderate depression of T cell activities are frequently found in patients with this condition. Both anergy on skin testing and depressed PHA responses are frequently seen.

4.2.5 Systemic Lupus Erythematosus

Depressed PHA responses are commonly found.

4.2.6 Liver Disease

Depressed PHA response and negative skin tests are frequently found in patients with advanced parenchymal disease of the liver, particularly that associated with chronic alcoholism.

4.2.7 Drugs

PHA response, and even skin test reactions, can be transiently supressed by a number of drugs including corticosteroids, cytotoxic drugs, acute ingestion of alcohol, and even under some circumstances, high doses of aspirin.

References

Catovsky, D.; Goldman, J.M.; Okos, A.; Frisch, B. and Galton, D.A.G.: T Lymphoblastic leukaemia. A distinct variant of acute leukaemia. British Medical Journal 2: 643-647 (1974).

Horwitz, D. and Lobo, D.T.: Characterization of the populations of human lymphocytes bearing easily detectable surface immunoglobulin. Journal of Clinical Investigation 56: 1464-1472 (1975).

Moretta, L.; Webb, S.R.; Gross, G.E.; Lydyard, P.M. and Cooper, M.D.: Functional analysis of two human T-cell subpopulations: help and suppression of B cell responses by T cells bearing receptors for IgM or IgG. Journal of Experimental Medicine 146: 184-200 (1977).

Wilson, J.D. and Nossal, G.J.V.: Identification of human T and B lymphocytes in normal peripheral blood and in chronic lymphocytic leukaemia. Lancet 2: 788-791 (1971).

Wilson, J.D.; Pang, G.T.M. and Baguley, D.M.: A differential effect of prednisone on human B and T lymphocytes. International Research Communication Service 2: 1690 (1974).

Chapter XVII

Neutrophil Function Tests

The major function of neutrophils is the ingestion or killing of invading micro-organisms, particularly bacteria. In order to achieve this the neutrophil passes through a series of activities. While these stages can be subdivided *in vitro, in vivo* they form a continuum.

As a first step towards killing micro-organisms, the neutrophil and micro-organism must come into contact. The directional movement of the neutrophil towards the organism is called chemotaxis. There are two aspects to chemotaxis: first, chemotactic factors must be released, and secondly the neutrophil must have the ability to recognise these factors and respond appropriately. As mentioned in chapter XI fragments of complement components are chemotactic, as are various tissue breakdown products and products of stimulated lymphocytes.

Having moved to the invading organism the neutrophil must then be able to recognise it as being foreign and thus worthy of ingestion. Coating of the micro-organism with recognition units is known as 'opsonisation', derived from the Greek word 'to prepare food for'. Opsonins are either antibody or complement components.

Ingestion follows rapidly upon a neutrophil's making contact with a suitably opsonised micro-organism and the final act in the drama begins with the metabolic activation of the neutrophil and the production of bactericidal products which leads to the destruction of the organism.

Failure of one or some of these mechanisms is associated with different disease states and commonly leads to syndromes of recurrent infection. This chapter describes in essence the tests of chemotactic, opsonic and neutrophil function that are commonly used for the investigation of patients with recurrent infections.

1. Chemotaxis

There are two aspects of chemotaxis, humoral and cellular. The first is concerned with the production of the chemotactic factor and the second the ability of a neutrophil to move towards a chemotactic factor. Very occasional cases have been described where the production of chemotactic factors from serum has been inadequate and this has generally been associated with complement deficiencies. Even more rarely the presence of an inhibitor of chemotaxis in the serum has been described. Abnormalities of neutrophil movement are found more commonly, though often in association with other diseases.

The physiological states and diseases in which deficiencies of neutrophil chemotaxis have been found are listed in table I.

1.1. Tests for Neutrophil Chemotaxis

There are two techniques commonly used to measure neutrophil chemotaxis. The first and most commonly used is the Boyden chamber. In this method, neutrophils are separated from a chemotactic solution by a filter. After a fixed length of time, the number of neutrophils migrating through the filter (usually expressed as

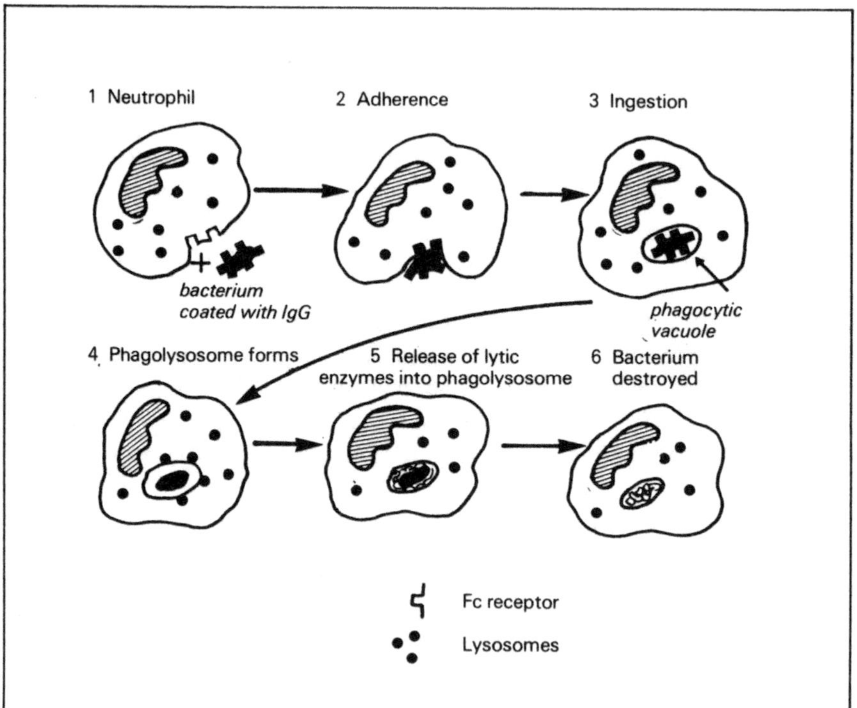

Fig. 1. The process of neutrophilic phagocytosis, showing actual intracellular destruction of a bacterium. Adapted from Thaler et al. (1977) with permission of the authors.

Table I. Deficiencies of neutrophil chemotaxis

Serum Factors
Complement deficiencies — Clr, C2, C3, C5
Agammaglobulinaemia
Circulating serum inhibitors
Intrinsic Neutrophil Defects
Neonatal life
Diabetes mellitus
Rheumatoid arthritis
Chediak-Higashi syndrome
Lazy-leucocyte syndrome
Drug treatment
— corticosteroids
— phenylbutazone

cells per high power field) is determined. A variation on this technique is to stop the fraction before the cells have passed through the filter and determine the depth to which leading cells have moved. The Boyden technique suffers from a number of technical problems so that before a diagnosis of chemotaxis deficiency is accepted the test should have shown similar results on repeated occasions.

An improved technique is being introduced to quantitate chemotaxis which involves placing a neutrophil suspension in wells in agar a short distance from another well containing chemotactic factor. This test is usually performed in plastic petri dishes and the neutrophils move under the agar towards the chemotactic containing well. The distance that the leading edge of a neutrophil reaches in a fixed time is a measure of the chemotactic ability of the neutrophil.

Both of these tests of chemotactic function are open to experimental variations which means that at present absolute values for chemotaxis cannot be adequately defined. The patient's results are expressed as a percentage of the controls done at the same time.

2. Opsonisation

Opsonins are proteins, principally antibody or complement, which facilitate phagocytosis. Thus measurement of the opsonic capability of serum depends upon methods of demonstrating phagocytosis

There are three levels at which phagocytosis can be determined and which, in theory, should give the same answer. Historically, the first method was to determine the number of particles or micro-organisms ingested, by examining the neutrophils microscopically. While time-consuming, this method is relatively simple using large particles like yeasts, but becomes very inaccurate with smaller particles like bacteria. The commonest particle used in this technique is baker's yeast because of its ready availability and visibility. Variations of the technique involve the use of radio-labelled micro-organisms to determine the proportion ingested. Endotoxin-coated lipid and latex particles have been used for this purpose.

The second level at which phagocytosis can be determined is to measure the removal of particles from neutrophil containing medium. Usually this is done by colony counts and has little to offer the routine laboratory.

The third group of techniques involves measuring the metabolic changes that take place in the neutrophil following phagocytosis. Methods have been described that utilise measurements of glucose oxidation, iodine fixation and reduction of the dye nitro-blue tetrazolium (NBT), following ingestion of particles.

None of the above ways of measuring the opsonic capacity of serum gives an absolute value that can be compared between laboratories. Again technical considerations mean that the measure can only be relative. Most laboratories doing tests of opsonic function will standardise the serum source used as a control by pooling serum from a number of normal donors. The patients' sera are then compared with the results obtained for the pooled normal sera.

Diseases in which opsonic deficiencies have been found include agammaglobulinaemia, C3 and C5 deficiency. Serum from the normal neonate has immature opsonic capacity.

3. Bacterial Killing by Neutrophils

The original technique used to determine bacterial killing by neutrophils was direct and measured the death of bacteria that had been ingested by the cells (or, at least, it measured the inability of bacteria to divide). This technique remains the cornerstone on which the diagnosis of a disorder of neutrophil-killing function must rest but, because of its expense and inconvenience, it is not a satisfactory screening method.

Other tests depend on the metabolic activation that takes place following ingestion of a micro-organism. These changes can be measured directly be determining the rate of production of radio-labelled CO_2 from radio-labelled glucose, or the production of superoxide ion, or, indirectly, by determining the reduction of the dye NBT to formazan, or the fixation of radioactive iodine to proteins.

The most common primary disease in which defective killing by neutrophils occurs is chronic granulomatous disease. The simplest test that can be used to exclude the diagnosis is the 'finger prick NBT'. In this test a drop of blood is incubated on a microscope slide. The granulocytes adhere to the glass and are activated. The clot is gently washed away and a drop of yellow NBT solution placed over the neutrophils.

Under normal circumstances blue formazan granules appear in the cytoplasm. This does not happen in chronic granulomatous disease. However, because of the serious implications of the disease confirmatory bacterial killing tests should be performed. Myeloperoxide deficiency is another rare cause of neutrophil dysfunction and its presence can be detected by histochemical staining of a blood smear.

References

Thaler, S.H.; Klausner, R.D. and Cohen, H.J.: Medical Immunology. (Lippincott, Philadelphia 1977).

Further Reading

Miller, M.E.: in Vyas, Stites and Brecker (Eds) Assays of Phagocytic Function in Laboratory Diagnosis of Immunologic Disorders, p.127-135. (Grune and Stratton, New York 1974).

Chapter XVIII

Acute Phase Proteins

Many diseases demonstrate an inflammatory process which involves plasma proteins termed acute phase proteins. Fluctuations in serum levels of these proteins are now being utilised to assess diseases which involve inflammation and tissue damage. They are a useful indicator in detection, diagnosis and treatment of such diseases.

Acute phase proteins are glycoproteins with diverse functions and varied electrophoretic properties. In this group of proteins are found carrier proteins for haemoglobin and copper, a protease inhibitor, a protein essential in clotting mechanisms and others whose properties are not as well defined. The proteins are sometimes considered to be divided into three main functional groups. The first two include transport and defence proteins which are secreted into the extracellular space where they fulfil their respective roles (Laurel, 1976). The third group contains those proteins described as passenger proteins and among these are numerous cellular proteins such as enzymes.

1. Types of Acute Phase Protein

1.1 Orosomucoid or α1-Acid Glycoprotein

The normal plasma concentration is 0.6 to 1.3g/litre. The biological properties of this protein are not well understood but its function is to inactivate progesterone and it is an acute phase reactant in response to inflammation. When measured immunologically it can be used as an indicator of tissue necrosis and inflammation.

1.2 α1-Antitrypsin or α1-Glycoprotein

The normal plasma concentration is 0.2 to 0.45g/litre. This protein is produced by hepatocytes and its biological function is to protect body tissues from autodigestion by trypsin, chymotrypsin and tissue enzymes that have trypsin-like activity. It has a particularly important role in protecting lung tissue from damage by endogenously released trypsin. There is significant leukocyte degradation in the lung and proteases, especially trypsin, are released into the lung. When there is a congenital α1-antitrypsin deficiency, juvenile emphysema can result because of lack of protection. α1-Antitrypsin is an acute phase protein reactant and increased levels are observed in acute infection, rheumatic disease, neoplasms, hepatitis, cirrhosis and in association with surgery. Decreased levels are seen in thyroiditis, pulmonary emphysema and juvenile cirrhosis. Secretion of α1-antitrypsin is under genetic control by Pi (protease inhibitor) genes and over 20 phenotypes have been identified. It is inherited as an autosomal recessive gene.

1.3 Caeruloplasmin

The normal plasma concentration is 0.2 to 0.4g/litre. This is an α2-globulin with an oxidase activity and is responsible for transporting copper. The concentration of caeruloplasmin is increased by oestrogen and because of this women who are pregnant, or patients on oestrogen therapy of any sort, show higher than normal levels. Increased levels are also seen in patients who have chronic infections, degenerative diseases, leukaemia, Hodgkin's disease, other malignant tumours, rheumatoid arthritis, or hyperthyroidism. Decreased levels are observed in newborn infants and patients with nephrosis. The main diagnostic significance is with the low levels seen in Wilson's disease (hepatolenticular degeneration) which is a familial condition where copper is deposited in the liver, kidney and lenticular nucleus of the brain.

1.4 Haptoglobin

The normal plasma concentration is 0.6 to 2.0g/litre. This is a haemoglobin-binding protein which has three genetically determined forms. It unites with haemoglobin forming haptoglobin-haemoglobin complexes. The haemoglobin is transported from the circulation back to the bone marrow and thus is a defensive system to prevent loss of iron after haemolysis. Haptoglobin also acts as an acute phase reactant. Increased levels are observed in inflammatory and degenerative disorders, neoplasms, nephrosis, rheumatic fever, acute pyogenic fevers and stress conditions. Low levels are seen in haemolytic anaemias, pernicious anaemia, hepatocellular disorders and mononucleosis.

1.5 Fibrinogen

The normal plasma concentration is 2.0 to 4.5g/litre. Fibrinogen is of primary importance as a clotting factor and is a fibrin precursor which is converted into fibrin by thrombin releasing a fibrinopeptide. It also acts as an acute phase reactant.

Increased levels are observed in many disease states. Low levels are seen in congenital afibrinogenaemia, acute fibrinogen deficiency and severe disseminated intravascular coagulation e.g. amniotic fluid embolus and cardiac prosthetic surgery.

1.6 C-Reactive Protein (CRP)

In healthy people CRP is usually absent but occasionally levels of up to 5mg/litre are found (Schultze and Heremans, 1966). The biological function of C-reactive protein is to promote phagocytosis. It also acts as an acute phase reactant. Increased levels are observed in pathological sera, acute rheumatism and acute stages of rheumatoid arthritis, infective hepatitis, bacterial and viral infections, malignancies, choleocystitis, myeloma and acute stages of tuberculosis. Newborn children born with inflammatory disease will show elevated CRP levels but maternal infections associated with elevated CRP levels will not be reflected in the neonate's serum.

2. Immunological Techniques used to Determine Levels of Acute Phase Proteins

Radial immunodiffusion and electroimmunodiffusion give precise and quantitative information of acute phase protein levels.

Electroimmunodiffusion is the preferred method for quantitative measurements because results can be obtained about 30 minutes after the sample has been taken. Radioimmunodiffusion can take anything from 6 to 24 hours. Utilising the electroimmunodiffusion method the physician is able to use acute phase phenomena in association with white blood cell and differential counts.

Formerly CRP was measured by a latex agglutination test and a precipitin test. Both these tests have now been superseded by the immunodiffusion techniques.

3. The Acute Phase Response

Acute phase proteins are produced in the liver and distributed by the hepatic circulation. An increase in synthesis rate is responsible for higher levels of acute phase proteins and although levels rise following inflammation there may be other modifying factors. Adrenal steroids may act as regulators and inhibitors and hormones such as insulin, and others, must be taken into consideration.

Overall the acute phase protein response is still not well understood although it has been suggested that these proteins may be a counteraction for lysosomal enzymes that are a product of necrosis and inflammation. The various time-concentrations of the acute phase proteins differ from protein to protein. Once tissue necrosis is present concentrations of CRP and α1-acid glycoprotein increase rapidly, in about 6 to 8 hours, and reach their maximum levels in between 48 and 72 hours. Increased levels of haptoglobin, caeruloplasmin and α1-antitrypsin appear after about 12 to 24 hours and reach their maximum between 72 and 96 hours. Elevated levels of CRP and α1-acid glycoprotein will be present as long as there is still tissue damage and levels of CRP give a close indication of the clinical course of the disease.

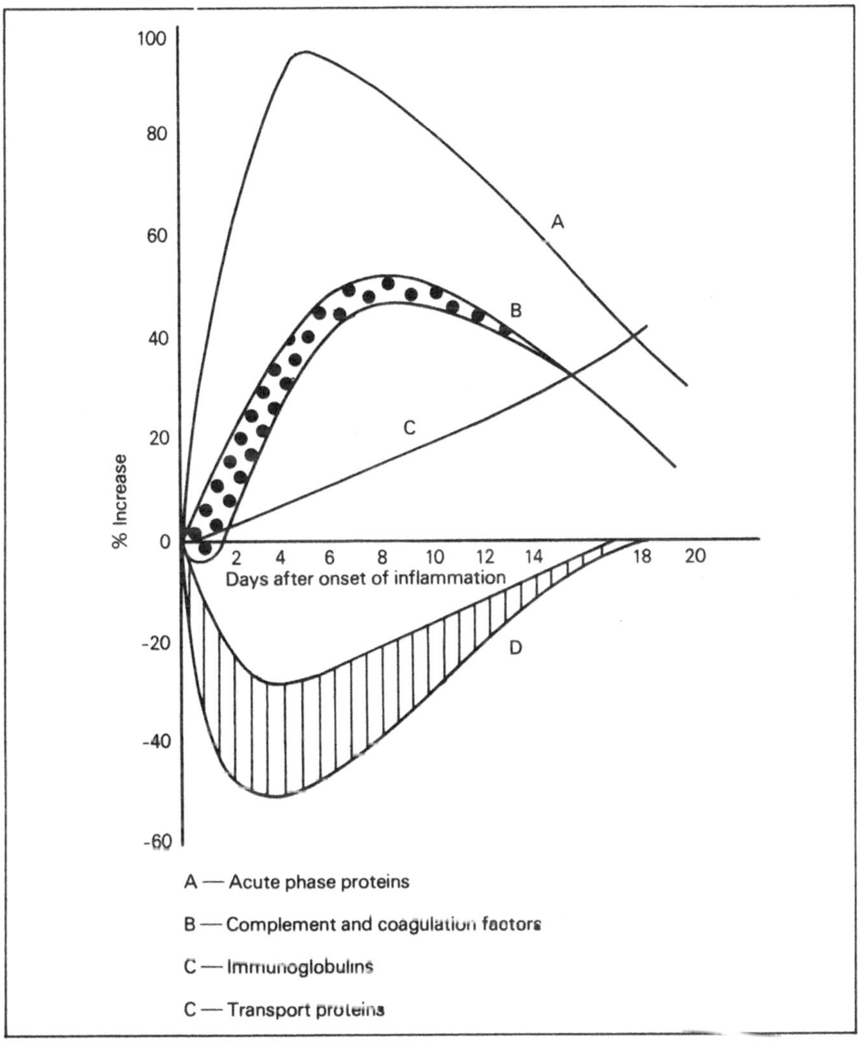

Fig. 1. The acute inflammatory protein response. From Laurell (1976) with permission of the author.

Haptoglobin, caeruloplasmin and $\alpha 1$-antitrypsin levels return to normal at a slower rate than CRP. Any prolonged elevation of acute phase proteins can be taken as an indication that the disease state is still present.

3.1 Use of Acute Phase Protein Levels in Diagnosis and Interpretation of Prognosis

Several general principles should be observed when results are interpreted.

1) Isolated or widely spaced measurements are of limited use because although the presence of inflammation can be detected by these determinations no diagnostic or prognostic information can be obtained. Serial determinations at suitable time intervals are needed to provide this type of information.

2) The determinations must be precise because small variations in levels can be of clinical importance and only properly quantitative methods give this accuracy.

3) A group of readings from several acute phase proteins is of more significance than readings taken of a single protein. Such a group could be $\alpha 1$-antitrypsin, haptoglobin and CRP.

3.2 Clinical Uses of Acute Phase Protein Levels

As mentioned above acute phase protein determinations can be used to establish the presence of an inflammatory process and the trends that the disease is following (fig. 1).

3.2.1 Post-surgery

Post-surgical patients can be checked for bacterial infection using acute phase protein levels which are more reliable indicators than white cell counts. The CRP and $\alpha 1$-acid glycoproteins should start to show a return to normal levels about the third day after surgery. If there is any increase in these acute phase protein levels after the fourth or fifth post-surgical day inflammation or tissue damage must be considered.

3.2.2 Rheumatic Diseases

Patients with rheumatic diseases can be monitored by acute phase protein levels rather than by ESR counts which can be affected by complicating factors.

3.2.3 Bacterial Infections

The highest levels of the 4 acute phase proteins normally studied are found in patients with bacterial infections.

3.2.4 Viral Infections

Usually these patients have relatively low levels of CRP and α1-acid glycoprotein but moderately elevated levels of α1-antitrypsin and haptoglobin.

3.2.5 Tumours

When tumours are associated with necrosis and inflammation the response pattern most commonly seen is a low CRP with a high elevation of α1-acid glycoprotein and moderate elevation of α1-antitrypsin and haptoglobin.

3.2.6 Myocardial Infarction

Here there is seen high CRP, low α1-acid glycoprotein and moderate elevation of haptoglobin and α1-antitrypsin levels.

It is most important to note that although these patterns can be considered typical of these disorders they are not diagnostic in themselves and must be considered along with all other relevant clinical criteria.

References

Laurell, C.B.: Determination and interpretation of plasma proteins. Australian Family Physician 6: 36-41 (1976).

Schultze, H.E. and Heremans, J.F.: Molecular Biology of Human Proteins, vol.1, p.149 (Elsevier, Amsterdam, 1966).

Further Reading

Hallen, J. and Laurell, C.B.: Plasma protein patterns in cirrhosis of the liver. Scandinavian Journal of Clinical and Laboratory Investigation 29 (Suppl. 124): 97-103 (1974).

Laurell, C.B.: The use of electroimmunoassay for determining specific proteins as a supplement to agarose gel electrophoresis. Journal of Clinical Pathology 28 (Suppl. 6): 22-26 (1974).

Chapter XIX

Tissue Typing

Histocompatibility is a measurement of surface antigens on cells from different individuals e.g. cells from a donor and a recipient. The ability of a graft to be accepted by a host shows that the donor and the recipient cells are histocompatible.

Histocompatibility antigens are present on the surface of most body cells, other than erythrocytes, and these antigens are analagous with the more well known erythrocyte surface antigens of the ASO and Rh systems. Human leucocyte antigens are made up of two polypeptide chains. The larger of the two is a glycoprotein (molecular weight 30,000) and this controls the antigenic specificity. The smaller chain (molecular weight 11,500) seems to be of the same structure as human β_2-microglobulin.

The histocompatibility system was first studied in the late 1950's and at this stage it was noted that patients who had received multiple transfusions and multiparous women both had leucoagglutinating antibodies in their sera (Dausset, 1954; Payne 1957). When sera were collected from this type of person and tested using leucoagglutination techniques it was found that they could be typed into various groups.

Periodic international workshops have been held and various investigators' trial sera have been tested with lymphocytes from common donors. Since 1965 there has been established a coordinating centre for the exchange of sera and this now holds a large number of typing sera (Hare et al., 1972). Protocols to be followed in assigning the various specificities of sera have been agreed on by a committee associated with the World Health Organisation and bulletins which list new specificities and protocols are published at regular intervals.

1. Genetics of the HLA Region

Human cells contain 46 chromosomes grouped as 23 pairs. One set of each pair is obtained from each parent. The chromosomes carry genes in the form of DNA and each gene is responsible for determining the structure of a specific protein polypeptide chain called the *gene product*, e.g. a histocompatibility antigen is determined by a gene specific for that particular antigen. The position of a gene on a chromosome is called the *gene locus* and when different genes occur at the same locus they are called *alleles*.

The human major histocompatibility system is a group of genes on the sixth chromosome (fig. 1). This region is thought to be approximately 1,000 genes long and is referred to as the HLA region. It is responsible for determining the structure of surface glycoproteins of all the cells in the body. These cell surface glycoproteins vary from individual to individual and because of differences in these antigenic determinants there is a major problem when tissue transplantation is performed between genetically non-identical patients.

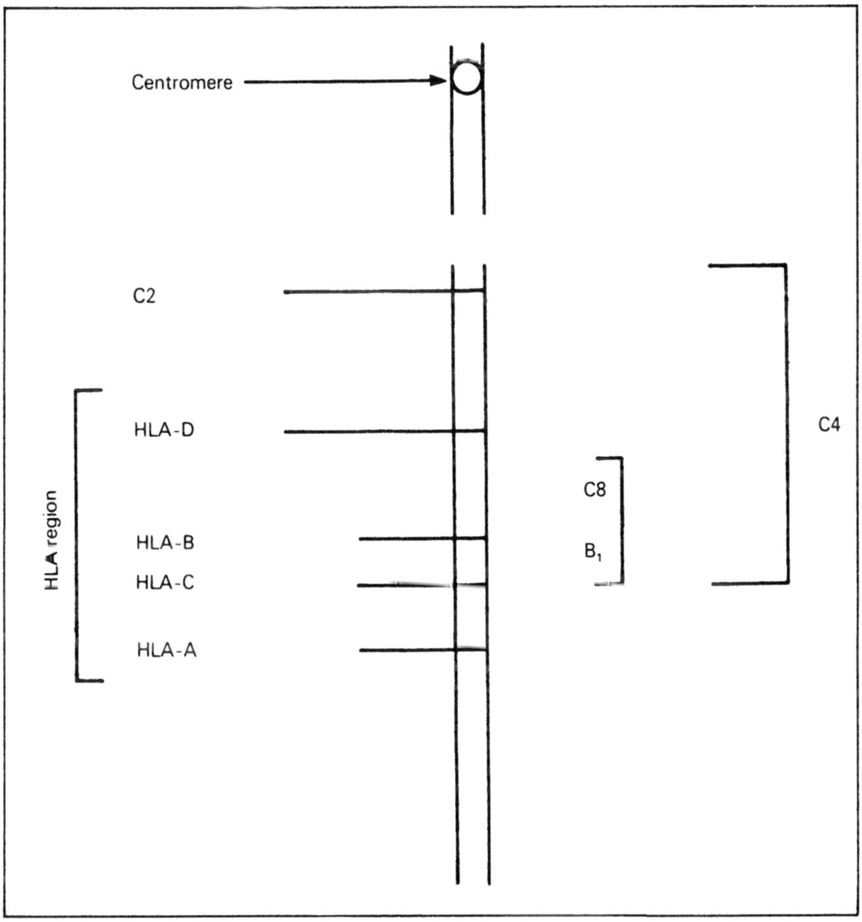

Fig. 1. Schematic diagram of the HLA system on human chromosome 6.

Within the HLA region lie four defined loci which are now termed HLA-A, HLA-B, HLA-C and HLA-D. The A, B and C loci determine antigens on the surface of all nucleated cells. The allelic genes at each locus determine their own set of antigens and these can be identified using available tested antisera.

HLA genes are *codominant* and therefore the antigen determinants inherited from both parents are expressed in the offspring.

The HLA system is also *polymorphic* which means that each HLA locus is multiallelic and an individual may have one of many alleles. It can be seen that the chance of finding complete HLA matching between any two unrelated people is remote.

It has been found that certain populations have a tendency to particular HLA specifications rarely found in other groups and anthropological studies of various inbred and isolated populations show a high incidence of certain gene frequencies in these groups.

2. Nomenclature of HLA Antigens

The International HLA workshops and World Health Organisation have established a nomenclature for the naming of the various HLA antigens (WHO Committee, 1975). Once an antigen has been clearly defined it is classified according to its locus, e.g. A, B, C etc., and it is then given an arabic number to further define it, e.g. HLA-A1. Those antigens that are as yet not clearly defined are written with a 'w' prefixed to the arabic numeral (table I). At the moment there are about 20 well characterised A locus antigens and about 25 B locus antigens (table II).

There have been a number of changes in nomeclature of the HLA antigens. Previously the A locus was termed LA, the B locus 4, the C locus AJ and the D locus was called MLR-S

3. Immune Functions Associated with Genes Close to the HLA Region

It has been found that genes closely located to the HLA region are able to control such functions as immune response and some phases of the complement system.

3.1 Immune Response Genes (Ir Genes)

These determine the degree of response an individual will show to a certain immunising antigen. These Ir genes affect T-cell function and it is thought that a protein which is found on the surface of B lymphocytes and macrophages (called immune associated antigen [Ia]) may be a product of these Ir genes.

Table I. The World Organisation notational scheme for HLA antigens. From WHO Terminology Committee (1975) with permission of the authors

HLA	A, B, C or D etc.	w (w)	1, 2 etc.
Region or system designation	Locus symbols	Symbol to indicate provisional specificity (may later be dropped when specificity is confirmed)	No. identifying specificities belonging to each locus

Table II. Known HLA antigens. Tables II to VIII adapted from Sasuzuki et al. (1977) with permission of the authors

A locus	B locus	C locus	D locus
A 1	B 5		
A 2	B 7		
A 3	B 8		
A 9	B 12		
A 10	B 13		
A 11	B 14		
A 28	B 18		
A 29	B 27		
Aw 23	Bw 15	Cw 1	Dw 1
Aw 24	Bw 16	Cw 2	Dw 2
Aw 25	Bw 17	Cw 3	Dw 3
Aw 26	Bw 21	Cw 4	Dw 4
Aw 30	Bw 22	Cw 5	Dw 5
Aw 31	Bw 35		Dw 6
Aw 32	Bw 37		
Aw 33	Bw 38		
Aw 36	Bw 39		
Aw 43	Bw 40		
	Bw 41		
	Bw 42		

3.2 Genes Associated with Complement Components

These have been found close to the HLA region. They include genes which determine properdin factor B and genes responsible for deficiency of the 2nd, 4th and 8th complement components.

4. Identification of HLA Antigens

4.1 A, B and C Locus

Antigens determined by the A, B and C loci are found on the surfaces of all nucleated cells (and on blood platelets). These antigens can be detected by serological techniques such as the lymphocyte cytotoxicity method. D locus antigens appear to be restricted to B lymphocytes.

Lymphocyte Cytotoxicity Method

In this test about 2000 viable lymphocytes are incubated for 1 to 2 hours with each of a chosen series of antisera. Fresh frozen rabbit serum is added as a source of complement. After incubation a vital dye is used to visualise the residual viable cells and the result used as an indication of the degree of antigen compatibility.

4.2 D Locus and Mixed Leucocyte Cultures (MLC)

At present the D locus antigens are just being recognised and the mixed leucocyte method is used to identify these antigens. Basically the test is as follows:

Lymphocytes from one individual (A) are cultured for several days with x-irradiated or mitomycin-C treated lymphocytes of a second individual (B). If B has D locus antigens that A does not, A's lymphocytes undergo transformation and the resulting DNA synthesis can be used as an index or response. B's lymphocytes do not undergo transformation because of the x-irradiation or mitomycin-C treatment.

Using individuals homozygous for D locus alleles it is possible to obtain typing cells which can then be used to test for the presence or absence of certain D locus alleles from other individuals.

5. Tissue Typing for Donor Selection

The main application of tissue typing has been in kidney and bone marrow grafting.

An ideal situation would be where only donors were used who were relatives with blood group ABO and HLA identical to the prospective recipient. However this criterion would restrict the choice to siblings of the recipient and even then the chance of the HLA system being identical would be only one in four.

HLA identity among siblings gives a reasonably good chance of a successful transplantation. Among HLA identical non-related individuals the success rate is considerably less but significantly greater than that between unmatched pairs.

Mixed lymphocyte reaction and graft rejections

Mixed lymphocyte reaction measurements in unrelated individuals have been found to give some indication of graft survival.

6. Specific Associations Between HLA and Disease

The first association noted between a disease and the HLA system was reported by Amiel in 1967. This was between an HLA-B locus antigen (then called 4C) and Hodgkin's disease. Since then a larger number of diseases have been reported to be associated with HLA-A, B and C antigens (Sasazuki et al., 1977). The most significant of these is the connection between B27 and ankylosing spondylitis and that between nasopharyngeal cancer and certain antigens.

In 1973 the first D locus antigen associated with a disease was reported — multiple sclerosis and Dw2.

Rapid progress has been made in analysing other HLA and disease associations although there must be some caution in accepting these results. Adequate control populations must be used, and other considerations such as racial background affect results.

The degree of association between HLA and disease can be measured according to relative risk and is calculated by the equation (RR = relative risk).

$$RR = \frac{\text{(no. of patients with HLA antigen) x (no. controls without the antigen)}}{\text{(No. of controls with antigen) x (no. of patients without the antigen)}}$$

At the time of writing approximately 40 diseases have been shown to be associated with HLA antigens.

6.1 Rheumatology

The association between ankylosing spondylitis and HLA-B27 is so pronounced that the presence of B27 can be used as a diagnostic aid very early in the development of this disease. More than 95% of Caucasian patients with ankylosing spondylitis have B27 compared to only 7 to 8% of controls. 50% of first degree relatives of B27 positive patients with ankylosing spondylitis have B27.

Reiter's syndrome also has a strong association with B27. People who experience reactive arthritis after infections such as *Yersinia enterocolitica* and Salmonella often have B27. See table III.

6.2 Neurology

Multiple sclerosis was initially associated with HLA-A_3 and later with B27 but latterly has been associated with HLA-Dw2. B8 has been connected with myasthenia gravis as has also Dw3. See table IV.

Table III. Rheumatological diseases associated with certain HLA antigens

Disease	HLA Antigen	Percent with antigen		Relative risk
		Patients	Controls	
Ankylosing spondylitis				
Caucasians	B27	95	8	87.8
Japanese	B27	67	0	305.7
Reiter's syndrome	B27	78	8	35.9
Yersinia arthritis	B27	79	9	24.3
Salmonella arthritis	B27	67	9	17.6
Psoriasis arthropathy	B27	42	8	7.1
(unspecified)	Bw17	25	8	3.9
Juvenile rheumatoid arthritis	B27	26	9	4.7
Rheumatoid arthritis	Dw4	36	16	3.0

Table IV. Neurological diseases associated with certain HLA antigens

Disease	HLA Antigen	Percent with antigen		Relative risk
		Patients	Controls	
Multiple sclerosis	A3	36	26	1.5
	B7	34	25	1.6
	Dw2	67	18	6.9
	Group 4[1]	84	33	
Myasthenia gravis	A1	45	26	2.5
	B8	52	23	4.4
Poliomyelitis	B7	38	19	2.6
Schizophrenia	A28	19	6	3.5
Manic depression	Bw16	13	5	2.5

1 Proposed B-cell alloantigen.

Table V. Dermatological diseases associated with certain HLA antigens

Disease	HLA Antigen	Percent with antigen		Relative risk
		Patients	Controls	
Psoriasis vulgaris	B13	20	5	4.7
	Bw17	26	8	5.0
	BW37	8	1	6.4
Psoriasis (unspecified)	B13	15	5	3.9
	Bw16	16	3	4.3
	Bw17	28	7	5.4
Psoriasis pustulosis	B27	28	9	3.8
Dermatitis herpetiformis	A1	69	30	4.4
	B8	77	25	9.2
	A10	39	13	3.1
Behcet's disease				
Caucasian	B5	35	11	4.3
Japanese	B5	75	31	6.5
Recrudescent herpes labialis	A1	56	25	3.7
	B8	33	17	2.5

Table VI. Endocrinology diseases associated with certain HLA antigens

Disease	HLA Antigen	Percent with antigen		Relative risk
		Patients	Controls	
Diabetes (juvenile onset insulin-dependent only)	B8	37	22	2.1
	Bw15	23	15	2.1
	Dw3	50	16	4.5
Thyrotoxicosis				
Caucasian	B8	42	24	2.5
Japanese	Bw35	67	21	5.0
Addison's disease	B8	50	23	3.9
	Dw3	70	18	10.5
Subacute thyroiditis	Bw35	77	13	22.2

Table VII. Gastroenterological diseases associated with certain HLA antigens

Disease	HLA Antigen	Percent with antigen		Relative risk
		patients	controls	
Chronic active hepatitis	A1	42	28	1.8
	B8	44	20	3.0
Idiopathic haemochromatosis	A3	78	27	9.5
	B14	26	3	9.2
Coeliac disease	A1	64	30	4.2
	B8	71	23	8.9
	Bw35	7	17	0.5
HB_sAg	Bw41	12	1	11.2
Pernicious anaemia	B7	36	22	2.2

Table VIII. Carcinomas associated with certain HLA antigens

Disease	HLA Antigen	Percent with antigen		Relative risk
		patients	controls	
Hodgkin's disease	A1	39	31	1.4
	B5	16	11	1.6
	B8	29	24	1.3
	B18	13	7	1.9
Acute lymphocytic leukaemia	A2	60	54	1.3
Retinoblastoma	B12	10	25	0.3
	Bw35	25	11	2.8
Nasopharyngeal cancer	Hs(Sr-2) B(Sin-2)	44	21	3.0

6.3 Dermatology

HLA-B Locus antigens have been associated with psoriasis vulgaris, and dermatitis herpetiformis has been connected with Dw3, B8 and A1. In this case the primary association may be with the B8 antigen and the other cases may be caused by a linkage disequilibrium between B8 and A1. See table V.

6.4 Endocrinology

When diabetes is of a juvenile onset and insulin-dependent it can be associated with both B8 and B5. People who have both these HLA factors have a much higher relative risk than those who have only one or other associated HLA factor. The two factors may have a cumulative effect and may affect susceptibility in this manner.

B8 is associated with thyrotoxicosis in people of Caucasian background but in Japanese patients Bw35 is the predisposing HLA factor. See table VI.

6.5 Gastroenterology

Chronic active hepatitis (CAH) is a type of liver disease which has been associated with both autoantibody formation and rheumatic complaints. It has been associated with both B8 and A1. This and other gastroenterological disease associations are listed in table VII.

6.6 Oncology

The association between Hodgkin's disease and an HLA antigen was the first reported. Among other malignant diseases (table VIII) retinoblastoma with its association with Bw35 shows the greatest relative risk.

6.7 Miscellaneous Diseases

Sjogren's syndrome has been associated with B8 and SLE with Bw13.

Conclusions

There are virtually no instances where the HLA type is 100% associated with a particular disease state; however there does definitely appear to be some predisposition to a number of diseases associated with particular genes of the HLA system, and it does seem that, in some cases, genetic factors may predispose to a particular disease.

References

Amiel, J.L.: Study of leucocyte phenotypes in Hodgkin's disease; in Curtoni, Mattiuz and Tosi (Eds) Histocompatibility Testing, p.79 (Munksgaard, Copenhagen 1967).

Dausset, J.: Leuco-agglutinins IV. Leucoagglutinins and blood transfusion. Vox Sanguinus 4: 190-198 (1954).

Hare, D.B.; Harris, C.E.; Kayhoe, D.E.; Ray, J.G. and Scott, R.C.: Catalogue of tissue typing antisera. Washington D.C.: DHEW Publication No. (NIH) 73-97: i-xvi, 1-941 (1972).

Payne, R.: Leucocyte agglutinins in human sera. Archives of Internal Medicine 99: 587-606 (1957).

Sasazuki, T.; McDevitt, H.O. and Grumet, M.D.: The association between genes in the major histocompatibility complex and disease susceptibility. Annual Reviews of Medicine 28: 425-452 (1977).

World Health Organisation—I.U.I.S. Terminology Committee: Nomenclature for factors of the HLA system. European Journal of Immunology 5: 889-891 (1975).

Further Reading

Amos, B.D. and Ward, F.E.: Immunogenetics of the HLA system. Physiological Reviews 55: 206-247 (1975).

Schaller, J.G. and Omenn, G.S.: The histocompatibility system and human disease. The Journal of Paediatrics 88: 913-925 (1976).

Chapter XX

Tests in Cancer

The presence of malignant tumours can sometimes be detected because of alterations in host immunity, such as generalised immune suppression, by an increase in some serum proteins, or by the demonstration of a specific host anti-tumour response. Despite considerable experimental work in this area there are only a few tests which have clear value in the diagnosis of cancer or in the monitoring of the progress of the disease.

1. Nonspecific Changes

A number of different tumours can produce the alterations described in this section.

1.1 Depressed Immunity

1.1.1 Immunoglobulins

In two situations serum immunoglobulins decline with the progression of tumours. Patients with multiple myeloma almost invariably show depressed immunoglobulins in the presence of a myeloma paraprotein. Some patients with lymphomas will similarly have low serum immunoglobulin levels. These occur most commonly in chronic lymphocytic leukaemia or in patients with non Hodgkin's lymphoma when initially, IgM, or IgM and IgA become depressed, and low IgG levels appear later in the disease. About 50% of patients with Hodgkin's disease show depressed IgM levels.

Patients with primary or secondary hypogammaglobulinaemia have a higher than normal incidence of tumours.

1.1.2 Cell-Mediated Immunity

Generalised depression of cell-mediated immune reactions is a common phenomenon in patients with lymphomas, particularly Hodgkin's disease. Testing for this can be carried out using a battery of recall antigens which measure the patient's delayed hypersensitivity skin reaction. This is described fully in chapter XIV (Skin Tests).

Anergy (non-responsiveness in delayed hypersensitivity skin tests) is observed more often in patients with Stages III and IV Hodgkin's disease than in patients with Stages I and II. About 50% of patients with non-Hodgkin's lymphoma will be anergic. The situation is less clear with other solid tumours. Over the age of 50, a clear association becomes apparent between the finding of anergy and the presence of a malignant tumour. The frequency of anergy is higher for some tumours than others, e.g. colonic carcinoma patients show pronounced immune depression while in patients with carcinoma of the breast the finding is uncommon.

A valuable application of this assay is in monitoring patients following treatment. Recovery of skin test reactivity in a patient formerly negative is a good prognostic sign. These tests can also be of assistance in the diagnosis of lymphomas or leukaemias of lymphoid origin. The use of lymphocyte function tests in malignant disease is reviewed in chapter XVI (Lymphocyte Function Tests).

1.2 Altered Serum Proteins

A number of nonspecific changes in serum proteins are commonly found in patients with cancer. The size of the tumour and the presence of necrosis, inflammation and infection each influence these changes. Some of these are discussed in the chapter on Acute Phase Proteins (page 122). C-reactive protein levels are frequently low while α1-acid glycoprotein, α1-antiprypsin, haptoglobins and complement (C3 and C4) are usually increased. IgA may be raised in tumours of the nasopharynx and gastrointestinal tract or uterus.

A higher incidence of autoantibodies, particularly smooth muscle antibodies, have been described by one group in patients with cancer.

2. Specific Antigen Changes Associated with Tumours

2.1 Paraproteins

These are fully discussed in chapter X (Immunoglobulins). Although not specific for multiple myeloma, they serve as a valuable and accurate marker for the progress of an individual patient's tumour.

2.2 Carcinoembryonic Antigen (CEA)

When first described by Gold and Friedman (1965), CEA was thought to provide a specific identification of colonic tumours. The antigen shared some determinants with fetal tissues, thus the name carcinoembryonic antigen. More recent evidence has shown that CEA is present in serum of patients with a variety of tumours and, at low concentration, in patients with a number of non-malignant diseases (Hansen et al., 1974).

CEA is measured by a radioimmunoassay. The concentration in serum of healthy people is usually below 2.5ng/ml. About 75% of patients with carcinomas of the colon, rectum, lung and stomach show CEA levels above 5ng/ml, patients with the more advanced and extensive tumours showing the highest levels. Raised levels are found in 50% of patients with tumours of breast, head, neck and uterus (Hansen et al., 1974).

Titres above 20ng/ml are almost always associated with metastatic tumours. Levels of greater than 100ng/ml can be found in association with extensive colorectal cancer.

False positive increased CEA levels occur with chronic bronchitis, emphysema and in patients who are smokers. Although the levels are rarely over 10ng/ml, this finding still reduces the diagnostic specificity of the assay.

A clear role for CEA is in monitoring the disease progress in patients following surgery. CEA levels should fall within 3 months of successful surgery for tumours and failure to do so, or a subsequent progressive rise, usually indicates continuing tumour growth.

2.3 Alphafetoprotein

This serum protein, an $\alpha 1$-globulin, is found at high concentration in serum of patients with hepatic cancer. It is also present early in fetal life.

In healthy adults the serum concentration is usually less than 30ng/ml. Very high levels, up to 12,000ng/ml, can be found in patients with liver cancer. Raised levels are also seen with teratoblastomas and in patients with acute hepatitis.

References

Gold, P. and Freedman, S.O.: Specific carcinoembryonic antigens of the human digestive system. Journal of Experimental Medicine. 122: 467-480 (1965).

Hansen, H.J.; Snyder, J.J.; Miller, E.; Vandervoorde, J.P.; Miller, O.N.; Hines, L.R. and Burns, J.J.: Carcinoembryonic antigen (CEA) assay. A laboratory adjuvant in the diagnosis and management of cancer. Human Pathology 5: 139-147 (1974).

Chapter XXI

Diagnosis of Immune Deficiency

Most of the assays discussed in the previous chapters measure the functional capacity of selected components of the immune system. Deficiencies of various parts of immunity may be congenital or acquired and these disorders are referred to as immune deficiency diseases. Although these diseases are uncommon, immunodeficient patients usually present with a common clinical problem, such as that of recurrent infections or infection with unusual organisms.

The symptoms listed in table I, in particular a history of recurrent infections, should raise suspicions of immune deficiency. Obviously it is important at first to exclude the more common causes of frequent infections before embarking on a detailed hunt for immune deficiency. Three questions must be considered:

1) Do the patient's circumstances provide sufficient explanation for recurrent or severe infections?

Children starting school, patients in circumstances with poor hygiene and debilitated patients all have sufficient reason for having increased infections.

2) Is the patient really suffering from recurrent infections or are symptoms and signs a result of some other mechanism such as allergy or asthma?

Recurrent upper respiratory symptoms, or recurrent cough may not represent infection at all but may be symptomatic of allergic rhinitis or asthma.

3) Are the patient's symptoms a manifestation of a generalised, non-immunological disorder such as diabetes, malignancy or renal disease?

In this case a full examination and appropriate tests depending upon the patient's signs and symptoms would be necessary.

If there is no obvious cause for the patient's infections (or other symptoms listed in table I) then immune deficiency must be considered a possibility. There are many forms of immune deficiency and they are classified as abnormalities of B lymphocytes (defective antibody production), T lymphocytes (defective cell-mediated immunity), phagocytes and complement. A full classification is found in tables II to IV. The more common conditions are briefly discussed below.

Table I. Clinical features associated with immunodeficiency. From Ammann and Wara (1975) with permission of the authors

1. *Frequently present, highly suspicious*
   a) Chronic infection
   b) Recurrent infection
   c) Unusual infecting agents
   d) Incomplete clearing between infections

2. *Frequently present, moderately suspicious*
   a) Skin rash (eczema, monilia)
   b) Diarrhoea (chronic)
   c) Growth failure
   d) Hepatosplenomegaly
   e) Recurrent abscesses
   f) Recurrent osteomyelitis

Table II. B Cell immunodeficiency diseases

Primary Immunodeficiency
X-linked hypogammaglobulinaemia (Bruton's)
Transient hypogammaglobulinaemia of infancy
X-linked hypogammaglobulinaemia with increased IgM
Selective IgA deficiency
Selective IgM deficiency
Selective deficiency of IgG subclasses

Secondary Immunodeficiency
Common variable immunodeficiency (acquired hypogammaglobulinaemia)
Chronic lymphocytic leukaemia
Myeloma

Table III. T Cell immunodeficiency diseases

Congenital thymic aplasia (Di George)

Chronic mucocutaneous candidiasis

Hodgkin's disease

Table IV. Combined T and B Cell immunodeficiency diseases

Severe combined immunodeficiency disease
Cellular immunodeficiency with abnormal Ig synthesis (Nezeloff syndrome)
Immunodeficiency with ataxia-telangiectasia
Immunodeficiency with eczema and thrombocytopenia (Wiskott-Aldrich syndrome)
Immunodeficiency with thymoma
Immunodeficiency with short-limbed dwarfism
Immunodeficiency with enzyme deficiency
Episodic lymphocytopenia with lymphotoxin
Cancer
Malnutrition

Various clinical features, such as age of onset of disease or nature of the infecting organisms, provide clues to the nature of the patient's immune defect.

1. Categories of Immune Deficiency (Amman and Wara, 1975)

1.1 B Lymphocyte Deficiency (Deficient Immunoglobulins)

Infections with *Pneumococci, Streptococci, Haemophilus, Pseudomonas, Meningococci,* and influenza are common. Patients have little problem with most viruses, fungi or other bacteria.

1.2 T Lymphocyte Deficiency

These patients are susceptible to infections with fungi, certain viruses (herpes and vaccinia), microbacteria, acid fast organisms and some low grade infections caused by intracellular bacteria such as *Listeria.*

1.3 Combined B and T Lymphocyte Deficiency

These patients develop infections in their first 3 to 4 months of life. The infecting organisms include fungi, viruses, *Pneumocystis* and atypical acid fast bacteria.

1.4 Phagocytic Abnormalities

Patients with these frequently present with local or systemic bacterial infections such as skin infections or osteomyelitis.

1.5 Complement Deficiencies

These patients frequently have SLE-like illnesses and increased susceptibility to bacterial infections.

2. Clinical Features of the More Common Immune Deficiency Disorders

2.1 X-linked Hypogammaglobulinaemia (Bruton's disease)

This rare condition affects boys only (Bruton, 1952). Patients lack B lymphocytes and plasma cells and produce little or no immunoglobulin. Symptoms of recurrent infections from common bacteria appear from about the age of 4 to 6 months after maternal IgG transferred across the placenta has decayed. Patients can suffer otitis media, bronchitis, pneumonia and meningitis.

Laboratory investigations show very low or absent gammaglobulins, and the total immunoglobulins are less than 2.5g/litre, with IgG less than 2.0g/litre and other Ig classes almost absent.

Long term management depends on gamma globulin replacement and antibiotics to treat infections.

2.2 Transient Hypogammaglobulinaemia of Infancy

Some children are late in initiating synthesis of their own immunoglobulins and become susceptible to bacterial infections from the age of 4 to 6 months until their own antibody levels rise at the age of about 12 to 18 months.

The diagnosis is made by determination of the child's immunoglobulins. IgG will be very low but significant levels of IgA and IgM may be present. B cells are normal. The condition is self limiting but infections are treated with antibiotics and gamma globulin replacement may be necessary.

2.3 Common, Variable, Unclassifiable Immunodeficiency (acquired Hypogammaglobulinaemia)

Patients with this disorder develop a gross deficiency of immunoglobulin production in childhood or adult life. It is not known why immunoglobulin synthesis fails. Patients develop recurrent pyogenic bacterial infections similar to those occurring in x-linked hypogammaglobulinaemia.

There is a high incidence of autoimmune disorders, such as rheumatoid arthritis, SLE, idiopathic thrombocytopenic purpura, dermatomyositis and haemolytic anaemia. Both males and females can be affected and the deficiency can develop at any age. Some patients also have some deficiency of cell-mediated (T cell) immunity.

Diagnosis depends on the history, exclusion of conditions such as leukaemia, myeloma and diabetes, and measurement of the patient's serum immunoglobulins. IgG is usually less than 2.0g/litre. Levels of IgM and IgA vary widely between patients and may be either absent or present in significant concentrations. B lymphocytes are present in normal numbers. *Management* consists of gammaglobulin replacement and the use of antibiotics when necessary.

2.4 Selective IgA Deficiency

This is the commonest form of immune deficiency and affects between 1:500 and 1:700 of the population (Schlegel and Kirkpatrick, 1978). The condition is sporadic but familial cases can occur. Most patients are asymptomatic but some present with recurrent sinopulmonary infections. Gastrointestinal disease, particularly coeliac disease, is relatively common in these patients. Autoimmune disorders, such as SLE and rheumatoid arthritis, and allergies occur frequently.

The *diagnosis* is made by demonstrating serum IgA levels of less than 0.1g/litre. Other immunoglobulin classes are normal.

Treatment is necessary only for the symptomatic patients and comprises antibiotic therapy for bacterial infections. Despite the fact that there is little IgA in gammaglobulin preparations some patients respond well to gammaglobulin replacement. As IgA deficient patients frequently have anti-immunoglobulin antibodies there is some hazard to this procedure.

2.5 Thymic Aplasia (Di George syndrome)

This rare condition results from congenital absence of a thymus. Children have an abnormal face and usually have hypoparathyroidism and congenital heart disease (Lischer and Di George, 1969). The diagnosis is made shortly after birth because of the patient's hypocalcaemia and susceptibility to infections as detailed above (1.2).

2.6 Mucocutaneous Candidiasis

Although this condition is rare in its most extensive form, mild cases are not uncommon. Patients have a selective susceptibility to infections with candida and present with infections in the mouth, nails, around the edges of their lips, and in severe cases, over much of their body. Many patients have associated endocrine defects. Iron deficiency is common.

The *diagnosis* is made by the clinical picture, demonstration of active candida infection and the patient's inability to generate a delayed hypersensitivity reaction to intradermal injections of candida. Various *in vitro* assays for T cell defects against candida can be conducted. *Management* consists of intensive local and, if necessary, systemic therapy with antifungal agents. Iron deficiency must be corrected and treatment with transfer factor or the immunopotentiating agent levamisole helps some patients.

2.7 Chronic Granulomatous Disease

Children with this disorder have a defect of leucocyte bactericidal function which renders them susceptible to chronic bacterial infections with pyogenic organisms such as *Staphylococcus aureus* and *S. epidermidis*. They develop lymphadenopathy, hepatosplenomegaly and chronic granulomatous skin infections.

The *diagnosis* is suggested by the history and confirmed by the nitroblue tetrazolium test where patients' leucocytes are found to lack the normal capacity to reduce a blue dye, nitroblue tetrazolium *in vitro*. Immunoglobulins and cell-mediated immunity are normal. *Management* is largely restricted to intensive antibiotic therapy. On occasions infusions of granulocytes can be helpful.

2.8 Defects of Phagocytosis

A host of defects have been described, some well characterised and others more ill-defined (Amman and Wara, 1975). The essential clinical picture is that of recurrent infections in patients with normal immunoglobulins. Details of tests are given in chapter X (Immunoglobulins). Management is by treatment of infections as they arise.

3. Investigations of Patients with Immune Deficiencies

A general laboratory screen should include full blood count and analysis of serum proteins, serum immunoglobulins and serum iron. At this stage the more common deficiencies will already have been detected. Neutropenia, hypogammaglobulinaemia, total iron saturation, will all come from this screen. If results are negative but a strong suspicion of immune deficiency remains, it is probably realistic to refer the patient to a specialist unit for further investigation.

Table V. Investigations for immune deficiency

1. *Evaluation of Humoral Immunity*
   a) Electrophoresis — gamma globulin
   b) Immunoelectrophoresis — semiquantitative
   c) Quantition of serum Ig — diffusion, nephelometry
   d) 1g sub-classes — specialist laboratory
   e) Isohaemagglutinins
   f) Antibody response to challenge
   g) *In vitro* Ig production

2. *Evaluation of Cell-Mediated Immunity*
   a) White cell differential count — lymphopenia
   b) Delayed hypersensitivity tests
   c) Lymphocyte populations
   d) Phytohaemagglutinin (PHA) response and mixed lymphocyte reaction
   e) Specific antigen stimulation
   f) Chest x-ray — thymus

3. *Neutrophil Function Assays*
   a) White cell differential count
   b) Chemotaxis
   c) Ingestion
   d) Nitro blue tetrazolium (NBT) test
   e) Neutrophil bactericidal assay

Table V summarises investigations which would be required for detection of deficiencies in each of the major groups described above. Full details of these assays are given elsewhere in the book and will not be considered further here.

Conclusions

Unfortunately a large number of patients with unexplained recurrent infections, or with infections caused by unusual organisms, will not prove to have immune deficiencies with the assay systems described above. This may be because the test systems used are not precise enough. For example, there are some people with recurrent respiratory tract infections who have a deficiency of one or other IgG subclasses and yet have normal levels of IgG overall. Secondly, some patients may have a defect of antibody against particular organisms and, unless this is assayed for, this too will not be detected. Thirdly, many people have recurrent infections because of local damage of particular anatomical sites, such as bronchiectasis, and under these circumstances obviously the cause of their repeated infections is not a deficiency in their immune function.

References

Amman, A.J. and Wara, D.W.: Evaluation of infants and children with recurrent infections. Current Problems in Pediatrics 5: 3-47 (1975).

Bruton, B.C.: Agammaglobulinaemia. Pediatrics 9: 722-728 (1952).

Lischer, H.W. and DiGeorge, A.M.: Role of the thymus in humoral immunity. Lancet 2: 1044-1049 (1969).

Schlegel, R.J. and Kirkpatrick, C.H.: Immune deficiency diseases; in Bellanti (Ed) Immunology II, p.644-689 (Saunders, Philadelphia 1978).

Further Reading

Ammann, A.J. and Hong, R.: Selective IgA deficiency: presentation of 30 cases and review of the literature. Medicine 50: 223-236 (1971).

Appendix

Summary of Immunological Tests Used in Diagnosis of Non-infectious Disease

The profile of immunological tests available for the diagnosis of infectious diseases has been discussed in Section I. In this appendix the tests of value in the diagnosis of non-infectious diseases are summarised, listed under the organs involved. This is not intended as a comprehensive list of all laboratory assays of clinical value; it is for use as a quick reference and is restricted to the tests discussed in the book.

Diseases of the Lung

Asthma

Whole blood count	eosinophilia common
Sputum	eosinophils common, Charcot-Leyden crystals
Skin tests (prick)	positive to range of inhalant allergens in atopic patients
IgE	raised in atopic patients

Extrinsic Allergic Alveolitis

Intradermal skin tests	late reaction after 5-8 hours
Precipitin tests for antibody to allergens such as Aspergillus	usually positive

Sarcoidosis

Electrophoresis	sometimes polyclonal gammopathy
Kveim skin tests	positive in 80% of cases
Delayed hypersensitivity skin tests	reduced or negative
Lymphocyte function tests	PHA response ↓

Skin Diseases

Atopic dermatitis (ezcema)

Skin tests (prick)	usually positive to wide range of allergens
Skin test (delayed hypersensitivity)	usually positive
Serum IgE	greatly ↑ in over 80% of cases

Contact Dermatitis

Skin test (patch test for 48 hours)	test for sensitising chemical produces positive reaction

Urticaria/Angio-oedema

Skin tests	usually negative and non-contributory. May be positive if urticaria induced by inhalant
Serum/complement	C3 or C4 usually normal if immune complexes are precipitating cause. C4 ↓ in hereditary angio-oedema
IgE	↑ with parasitic infections
Eosinophils	↑ with parasitic infections

Mucocutaneous Candidiasis

Skin tests (delayed hypersensitivity)	negative to Candida but may be positive to other antigens
Lymphocyte function tests	positive reaction to Candida *in vitro*

Diseases of the Joints

Rheumatoid Arthritis

Special investigations	
Examination of synovial fluid for cells and complement	neutrophils ↑ complement ↓
Immunological tests	
Rheumatoid factor (Rose Waaler, RF latex)	positive in 75% cases
Antinuclear antibody	positive in 20-50% of cases
LE cells	positive in 20% of cases
Biological false positive for syphilis	true in 10% of cases
Serum/complement (C3, C4)	normal in 90% ↓ in 10% of cases
Cryoglobulins	positive in 5-10% of cases
Acute phase proteins	↑ in most cases

Juvenile Rheumatoid Arthritis

Special investigations	
Examination of synovial fluid for cells and complement	neutrophils ↑ complement ↓
Immunological tests	
Rheumatoid factor (Rose Waaler, RF latex)	positive in 10% of cases
Antinuclear antibody	positive in 10% of cases
LE cells	positive occasionally
Serum/complement (C3, C4)	normal
Acute phase proteins	↑ in active disease
ASO	↑ in 20-30% of cases

Ankylosing Spondylitis

Rheumatoid factor (Rose Waaler, RF latex)	negative
Antinuclear antibody	negative
Serum/complement	normal
HLA antigen	B27 in 95% of cases

Reiter's Syndrome

Special investigations

Examination of synovial fluid	neutrophils ↑

Immunological tests

Rheumatoid factor (Rose Waaler, RF latex)	usually negative
Serum/complement (C3, C4)	normal

Multi-System Diseases

Systemic Lupus Erythematosus (SLE)

Rheumatoid factor (Rose Waaler, RF latex)	positive in 30% of cases
Antinuclear antibodies	positive in 95-100%
LE cells	positive in 70-80% of cases
Biological false positive for syphilis	positive in 10-20% of cases
Serum/complement (C3, C4)	↓ in active disease
Acute phase proteins	↑ in active disease
Autoantibodies	thyroid autoantibodies positive in 20% of cases
Anti double-stranded DNA antibodies	found in most patients at some stage of their disease
Serum electrophoresis	gammaglobulins usually ↑

Sjogren's Syndrome

Rheumatoid factor (Rose Waaler, RF latex)	Rose Waaler positive in 70% of cases RF latex positive in 90% of cases
Antinuclear antibody	positive in 70% of cases
LE cells	positive in 20% of cases
Autoantibodies	salivary gland positive in 50% of cases
Anti double-stranded DNA antibodies	rare
Serum electrophoresis	gammaglobulins raised in 50% of cases

Progressive Systemic Sclerosis (Scleroderma)

Rheumatoid factor (Rose Waaler, RF latex)	positive in 25% of cases
Antinuclear antibody	positive in 70% of cases (often speckled or nucleolar pattern)
Serum/complement (C3, C4)	normal
Autoantibodies	anti RNA antibodies common, extractable nuclear antigens antibodies usually negative
Anti double-stranded DNA antibodies	rare
Serum electrophoresis	gammaglobulins raised with active disease

Diseases of Gastrointestinal Tract or Liver

Chronic Atrophic Gastritis/Pernicious Anaemia

Parietal cell antibodies	usually present (> 90%)
Intrinsic factor antibodies	appear with the development of pernicious anaemia
Thyroid autoantibodies	common

Acute Hepatitis

HB Ag	appears at variable times during infection; identifies hepatitis B
HB Ab	signals recovery phase
Serum electrophoresis	polyclonal gammopathy
Acute phase proteins	raised
Smooth muscle antibodies	appear in up to 80% of patients with hepatitis A or B
Complement	sometimes ↓ from depressed synthesis
Cell-mediated immunity	usually depressed

Chronic Acute Hepatitis

Smooth muscle antibodies	positive in most patients
Serum electrophoresis	polyclonal gammopathy
Mitochondrial antibodies	often positive
HB Ag and Ab	in 25% of very aggressive cases
IgM and IgA	↑ 75% of cases
Antinuclear antibody	up to 50% of cases
LE cells	occasionally
Complement	often depressed

Primary Biliary Cirrhosis

IgM	usually ↑
Mitochondrial Ab	positive in 90% of cases — rare in other conditions
Acute phase proteins	raised in most patients
Electrophoresis	diffuse gammaglobulins
HB Ag	positive in 20-30% of cases

Heart Disease

Rheumatic Fever

Standard tests

Whole blood count	Hb commonly ↓ and WBC ↑ almost all cases ESR
Urinalysis	normal. RBC transiently in few patients
Throat swab	may culture Group A B haemolytic streptococcus

Immunological tests

ASO AHT ASK Anti DNase B	individually raised in 60-70% of cases. With battery of tests 1 or more raised in 95-98% of cases
Serum electrophoresis	diffuse ↑ alpha and gammaglobulin
Serum/complement (C3, C4)	normal or ↑
Acute phase proteins	↑ in almost all cases

Renal Diseases

Acute Post Streptococcal Glomerulonephritis

Standard tests

Whole blood count	Hb ↓ WBC ↑ ESR ↑
Urinalysis	RBC, red cell casts

Immunological tests

ASO ASK AHT Anti DNase B	individually raised in 60-70% of cases. With battery of tests 1 or more raised in 95-98% of cases
Serum electrophoresis	diffuse ↑ gammaglobulins
Serum/complement	C3 very low, C4 normal or ↓ CH50 very low, C3 nephritic factor activity often present
Acute phase proteins	raised

Endocrine Diseases

Hyperthyroidism

Thyroid microsomal antibodies	present in 80-90% of cases
Thyroglobulin antibodies	present in 30-60% of cases
Parietal cell antibodies	present in 30-35% of cases

Hypothyroidism

Thyroid microsomal antibodies	present in 80-90% of cases
Thyroglobulin antibodies	present in 40-60% of cases

Primary hypoadrenalism

Antiadrenal antibodies	50% of patients

Diabetes Mellitus

Anti islet cell antibodies	common in juvenile onset diabetes, rare in others

Other autoantibodies

Thyroid microsomal, Thyroglobulin PCA	all occur with increased frequency

Key to Abbreviations

ADCC	Antibody-dependent cell cytotoxicity
AHT	antihyaluronidase test
ALL	acute lymphocytic leukaemia
AGN	acute glomerulonephritis
AMA	antimitochondrial antibodies
ANA	antinuclear antibodies
ASK	antistreptokinase
ASO	antistreptolysin-0
C1-9	complement components
CAH	chronic active hepatitis
CEA	carcinoembryonic antigen
CFT	complement fixation test
CLL	chronic lymphocytic leukaemia
CRP	C-reactive protein
DNA	deoxyribonucleic acid
DNCB	dinitrochlorobenzene
DT	dye exclusion test
ELIZA	enzyme-linked immunosorbent assay
ENA	extractable nuclear antigens
FAT	fluorescent antibody test
FTA-ABS	fluorescent treponemal antibody absorption
HAT	haemagglutination test
HAV	hepatitis A virus
HBsAg	hepatitis B surface antigen
HBV	hepatitis B virus
HLA	histocompatibility system
IgA, M etc	immunoglobulin A etc
Ir genes	immune response genes
LAT	latex agglutination test
LATS	long acting thyroid stimulator
LATS-P	LATS protector
MLC	mixed leucocyte cultures
NBT	nitro-blue tetrazolium
PCA	parietal cell antibodies
PHA	phytohaemagglutinin
PPD	purified protein derivative
RAST	Radioallergosorbent test
RCFT	Reiter complement fixation test
RF	rheumatoid factor
RPR	rapid plasma reagin
SCAT	sheep cell agglutination test
SIg	surface immunoglobulin
SKSD	streptokinase-streptodornase
SLE	systemic lupus erythematosus
SMA	smooth muscle antibody
SRBD	sheep red blood cell
TEC	total eosinophil count
TPHA	T. Pallidum haemagglutination
TPI	T. Pallidum immobilisation
VDRL	venereal disease research laboratory
WR	Wasserman reaction

Subject Index

G

H

I

U

V

W

X

Y

GPSR Compliance

The European Union's (EU) General Product Safety Regulation (GPSR) is a set of rules that requires consumer products to be safe and our obligations to ensure this.

If you have any concerns about our products, you can contact us on ProductSafety@springernature.com

In case Publisher is established outside the EU, the EU authorized representative is:

Springer Nature Customer Service Center GmbH
Europaplatz 3
69115 Heidelberg, Germany

Batch number: 10584556

Printed by Printforce, the Netherlands